CHANGE YOUR SPACE

*Reclaim Your Home,
Your Time
and Your Mind*

by Dilly Carter

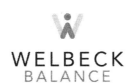

WELBECK
BALANCE

Published in 2023 by Welbeck Balance
An imprint of Welbeck Non-Fiction Limited

Part of Welbeck Publishing Group

Offices in: London – 20 Mortimer Street,
London W1T 3JW &
Sydney – 205 Commonwealth Street,
Surry Hills 2010

www.welbeckpublishing.com

Design and layout
© Welbeck Non-Fiction Ltd 2023
Text © Dilly Carter 2023

A CIP catalogue record for this book is
available from the British Library.

ISBN 978-1-80129-285-6

Internal design by Goldust Design

Printed in Great Britain by
CPI Group (UK) Ltd, Croydon CR0 4YY

10 9 8 7 6 5 4 3 2

MIX
Paper | Supporting
responsible forestry
FSC
www.fsc.org
FSC® C171272

Note/Disclaimer

To Charley and Nelly

About Dilly

Dilly Carter is a master in detoxing space; a straight-talking and practical professional organiser who believes that if we all cut the clutter, we will enjoy life more. She is the founder of Declutter Dollies (@declutterdollies), an organising and home-styling service. She provides decluttering advice on BBC One's *Sort Your Life Out*.

CONTENTS

INTRODUCTION

Do you feel you are stuck in a rut with your home?

Are you fed up with how it functions?

Do you want to gain back control?

Are you ready to live a clearer, calmer, more organised life?

Have you realised that change is the only thing you need to commit to?

If the answer to these questions is 'yes', then it's time to change your space, to declutter your home. Decluttering will not only give you an orderly living space, but it will also lead to an improvement in the way your home functions day to day *and* it will help to clear your mind. Once you know where your belongings are and that you have only what you really need, your daily routine will be smoother, you'll feel calmer and more in control, and the benefits of having a tidy physical space will be mirrored in your mental health.

Change is inevitable. At some point, we will all experience life-changing events: a birth, a marriage, death, and possibly a separation or a divorce. Along with these big changes we also experience personal growth, and these life shifts mean we often then need to change our living

Clearing your space will lead to an improvement in the way your home functions day to day AND it will help to clear your mind.

space too. But how you deal with this is vital – and that is why I've written this book to guide you.

My working life as a professional organiser reflects my ethos of living a life unhindered by *stuff*. Alongside my Instagram account @declutterdollies, you might have spotted me on TV sharing organising tips on *Lorraine* or decluttering family homes on the BBC's *Sort Your Life Out*. I've done this job for nearly 20 years and have worked in a variety of private homes across the world.

In this book, my mission is to share the benefits of decluttering so that you too can reclaim your home, your time and your mind.

Every time I look out of my window, I see the annexe where my mum now lives. Seeing her there is a constant reminder of what a life surrounded by too much clutter can do to your mental health. It also reminds me of how I don't want to live my life. When I finished writing my first book, *Create Space*, my mum was just moving out of the house I share with my husband Charley and daughter Nelly-Reet to start afresh in her own space – in the annexe we built for her. My mum has bipolar disorder and having her own personal space has seen her mental health improve so much that she no longer needs full-time care. She's more self-sufficient than ever. She's also living with less – less stuff and less clutter.

My mum's bipolar disorder overshadowed much of my early life. I spent my teenage years frequently visiting her in a psychiatric hospital; the trauma and darkness I saw in that place will never leave me. People breaking their doors... rocking on beds wrapped up in old blankets... rooms with nothing more than a metal bed frame and a mattress... It was a very cold, very scary place to be in, especially when you're only 11 years old. I was just a child but even I could see that there was a link between a person's physical environment and their mind, which I think is what has made me so incredibly aware of the importance of the spaces we live in.

By restricting the patients' belongings, it seemed that the hospital also restricted their personality. Even in a prison cell you're able to bring some identity the walls. But in that stark hospital environment, it felt like everyone was just a number in a box, with nothing but their minds to occupy them. Every person in that institution seemed to have been stripped of their identity, their *humanity*, and reduced to a physical shell.

At home, we lived surrounded by my parents' clutter and that chaos did have a detrimental effect; but having all her possessions taken away was equally damaging to my mother's state of mind.

I realised that the space – the environment – around her was key to my mother's wellbeing.

It makes a huge difference living minimally compared to having a house full of items that you don't love. But I've also seen the results of living with nothing, so even though I prefer to live with less, I believe people always need to have some personal belongings around them to give them purpose and make them happy. You just need to find a balance between clutter and comfort.

I grew up in Shepperton, Middlesex. Throughout my teens, because my dad was so focused on his work as a chartered accountant and my mum was in and out of hospital, my house became the party house, the hangout house. There were never any parents there! But as well as spending loads of time with my friends, I also took on my mum's role, in that I looked after my dad. We had support from our neighbours, but because my dad could only just about put bread in the toaster, I cooked for him. When I was 18, my parents moved to Somerset and I also left our family home. Once they had moved and stopped working, my dad was diagnosed with dementia. He spent his last years in a care home; I think he worked so hard that it probably caused his illness.

It was 10 years ago that we hit a crunch point and I knew I had to rescue my mum from living alone. After my dad passed away, I had been working hard and travelled to America, Canada and Australia with Charley (my then-boyfriend, now-husband!). While I was away, Mum and I exchanged regular emails and it seemed like she was fine, but I hadn't seen her in person – or visited the house – for two years. Charley and I got married and had our and I got married and had our honeymoon in Bali. When I returned to the UK, I found my mum living in a state of total disarray. While I had been away, my mum had been living alone and her mental health had declined. Her disordered mental state had led to the house becoming beyond cluttered – it was out of control, mirroring her internal state. I realised something had to be done.

Before I even walked through the door, I could see piles of unopened mail on the doormat, and looking through the windows to the front room there seemed to be even more unopened mail. Inside, I was met with utter chaos. There were stacks of papers on the floor and only one little empty patch on the sofa where she could just about perch to watch TV. Her desk next to her bed was also covered with papers (as well as cat hair). The kitchen surfaces were cluttered with an array of pans – some clean, some dirty – and, apart from out-of-date food, there was barely anything to eat in the house.

As I started to clear out the clutter, I saw that what was once just an untidy house had become something beyond my mum's control. As I cleared out more, it got worse... I discovered bags upon bags full of

iTunes gift vouchers, MoneyGram receipts and Western Union receipts. It became clear that she had been a victim of numerous scams. She was vulnerable and alone, and criminals had taken advantage – calling her landline many times a day, building relationships with her and convincing her to share gift codes or transfer money to various different accounts. She had been sending £50, £100, £200 at a time, wiping out her savings. There were also boxes of pills – vitamins, diet pills, all things that she didn't need. If there was a cold caller at the door, she would buy whatever they were selling. We worked out that she had lost nearly £50,000... It's horrifying to think that people would prey on an elderly lady, especially someone so vulnerable. I'd seen my mum live as a prisoner to her mental health for many years, but seeing her a prisoner to the clutter in her own home was the lowest of the lows. The combination of the physical mess and my mum's health situation was completely overwhelming.

As well as physically clearing out her home, it was clear that I needed to take control of her life to make things better. At the time, I was already working as an organiser in private homes, so I knew I could get my mum's house into better shape. I took pictures of the 'before' and had a vision of how it *should* look, and spent the next weekend decluttering, getting rid of all the stuff she didn't need, tidying and arranging. I knew that by clearing the space she could have a more positive state of mind. I'd seen it so many times when I'd worked with my private clients.

When you have order in your house, it instantly helps to improve your mood.

It's the little changes that often make the most difference: changing the time on the oven clock to the correct one, cleaning the bedroom mirrors or making the bed. These small changes are the things that always make clients smile and say, 'I can't believe you did that! Thank you so much!' So I knew that the bigger task of completely clearing my mum's house would help her immeasurably.

Even *during* the process of clearing out the clutter, I could see it was already improving my mum's mood. Every time she came back into one of the rooms I'd been working on, you could see the delight on her face as she saw the space I'd cleaned and the changes I'd made. As the surfaces were cleared, my mum's attitude transformed and I saw the light come back into her eyes. I knew that once I'd decluttered the space, she would be able to keep on top of it, with my help. When you're at the lowest point, having someone to help can make it easier to climb back up.

With my mum, changing her space allowed her to temporarily reclaim her home, her time and her own mind, but her mental health history meant that we knew it may not be a change that could be sustained. It would need constant revisiting, so we made the decision that it was time for us to take over her care. Eventually my mum moved into our home, although it wasn't an immediate change. We had to sell her house and then find ourselves a new house big enough for us all to live in. In this period of waiting, we welcomed our daughter Nelly in 2013. It wasn't until 2015 that my mum moved in. We had a tiny two-bed house – she lived in the spare room and we shared our limited space.

We have lived together as a multigenerational household for eight years now. It's been a time of big changes for us all, but Mum is finally settled and we have reached a place of calm as a family. The only way we have been able to do this is by living clutter-free, which has allowed us to move forward into the next steps in our lives together.

HOW YOUR SPACE IMPACTS YOUR LIFE AND STATE OF MIND

The space you live in can become a mirror of your life and your emotions.

Clearly, there was a link between the chaos at my mum's house and her bipolar disorder. It's an extreme example, but in my job I've seen homes that belong to people who are not diagnosed with mental health issues and are still chaotic, and that mess can impact *anyone's* mood. As I've built my business over the last 20 years, sharing before-and-after shots of decluttered cupboards and refreshed rooms on Facebook and Instagram, I've seen that everyone has a different take on what is an acceptable level of clutter. *How* that clutter affects each of us is different too.

Whether you are an extreme case, where the volume of your possessions is severely impacting your ability to get by on a daily basis, or you're someone who feels overwhelmed by a lack of storage and doesn't have a clue where to start to tidy it all up, this book will take you back to the crux of *why* you're in this situation, as well as dealing with the practical details (like working out how to have enough storage for your things, how to start your decluttering journey and how to make your life smoother). I will guide you to think about why you've arrived at this situation so that you can get yourself out of it and never make those mistakes again. I hope that you will find some take-aways from this book that help you to get to a place of calm.

HOW YOUR SPACE NEEDS TO CHANGE AS YOU/ YOUR LIFE CHANGES

Perhaps you are faced with thinking about a big change in your life and wondering how to handle it. Everyone's lives are in a constant state of flux, whether we like it or not. Change is often the catalyst for things going slightly wrong and for allowing the clutter in our homes to get on top of us. You might be welcoming a baby, adopting a child, or having to make space to care for an elderly relative. Perhaps you've had to downsize (or even upsize), you're moving to university, moving back in with parents, going through a divorce, or inheriting a space.

The key to making these types of changes work is to be flexible, because this will help you stay in control.

It's also key to have every family member involved, if you can. Mum never dreamed of living at the bottom of my garden when she was 82 and it wasn't in my life plan (let alone Charley's!) to be living with a parent as a newlywed; however, we made it work by being flexible and respecting each other's needs.

My experience with my mum's mental illness is the reason I'm here today. It's also the reason I'm the perfect person to talk you through your own decluttering process. Not only can I advise you about what you need to change in your house, I know *why* you need to change it, because I'm still doing it. I'm living it, breathing it every single day.

I am here to give you real life, real homes and real talk. If you're reading this book, it's likely that you will have realised that you need to change, or perhaps you're about to enter a new stage in your life with which you need help.

What is the feeling that you want to try and create in your space?

This book will guide you through all the stages of decluttering, organising and dealing with change. It all starts with working out what matters to you and deciding what you actually need in your home.

Ask yourself some key questions: What do *you* need as a person? What makes you happy? Is it 40 pairs of shoes? I know that owning 40 pairs of shoes might make some people happy – and that's fine – but you need to make sure that those shoes don't impact anyone else in your home. Always ask yourself what you see as more valuable: is it having the shoes or the physical space that they take up (and the mental release from not having to tidy them up!)? Perhaps you might be happiest just feeling comfortable in the space that you're living in. Do you want to be able to sit on the sofa, happily relaxing, watching TV, and not be surrounded – overwhelmed – by stuff? What is the feeling that you want to try and create in your space?

Through the pages of this book, I will teach you the benefits of changing your space and valuing what you already have (while avoiding the pitfall of accumulating more).

HOW TO USE THIS BOOK

Being organised is not just about decanting your cereals into matching containers.

I never want you to feel that a 'look' is what we are striving for. Of course I want to make your home look beautifully organised and chic, but it's vital that you understand that being in control and on top of your house is much more important than having an Instagrammable aesthetic.

Change Your Space is divided into five sections:

> **ADAPT Your Space**

> **SHARE Your Space**

> **CHANGE Your View**

> **ACCEPT Your Situation**

> **CHALLENGE Yourself**

I've divided this book into these chapters because they follow the process you will need to go through to successfully change your space.

The first two sections are about physical changes, while the chapters on changing and accepting are more led by your mindset.

On a personal level, these are the stages I've gone through myself (and in this order). When you don't know where to start, following this structure will help you. When you identify how you need to adapt to change, it will give you the practical know-how to share your space. So many of us experience change unexpectedly, or for reasons that are out of our control, but whenever I've known that there has to be a change, I then move on to accepting that change.

Each section is led by a key moment that shaped my life, which echoes the theme of the chapter, and I share the lessons I've learned from the homes I've organised, too. Each explains why following my suggestions for decluttering and clearing will help your wellbeing, as well as showing you just how beneficial those changes can be. There is a key tidying idea to help you do some practical work, motivational pointers with things to aim for, and inspiring quotes along the way. I'm always totally honest about the work you need to do and the hard questions you need to ask yourself, and I am

here to guide you through realistic methods to create a vision that will inspire your decluttering plans.

The first four sections of the book also correspond with the seasons. Working with the seasons is a great way to regularly remind yourself to reset and to help you keep on top of any clutter that might be creeping into your space.

Each season, I'll guide you through two large spaces in your house that you can declutter, along with two smaller areas that could benefit from a Dolly Dash.

'Dolly Dash' is my name for a fast, timed tidy-up. The reason we do Dolly Dashes is so you can see results in such a short time! They help motivate you on your tidying journey.

Removing clutter improves your mood immeasurably and when you've broken a bad habit, you've made a big win. Even a little win is such a mood-booster.

In the last section of the book, CHALLENGE Yourself, you'll find the 30 Days of Change Challenge that will help you declutter your home. I'd love you to take up this challenge.

In line with the changing seasons, I have also included a 7-day challenge for each season. Please join in!

There are also some resources and training material, plus a useful planner to help you tackle the main rooms in your house. But before you get started, check out my 6 Golden Rules of Decluttering below. (Write them out and stick them on the fridge!)

MY 6 GOLDEN RULES OF DECLUTTERING

Every time you approach a space or room to tidy or declutter, I want you to go through each of these steps in order. Stick to them and tidying and decluttering will become second nature!

1. **Assess** – what do you need to change/what would you like to change?

2. **Clear** – always clear the space entirely

3. **Group** – put items together that need to be together

4. **Categorise** – allocate items to the right places (e.g. garage items in the garage, etc.)

5. **Storage** – choose the correct type of storage for each group of items

6. **Label** – make sure you know what is where

GETTING STARTED

It's so important to understand that decluttering is not a 'one and done' process. People will moan, 'Well, I've done it – but I feel like I'm constantly doing it.' Yet life is continuously moving; we all experience small daily changes, as well as some really big life changes, not to mention the regular seasonal shifts we live through.

Therefore, it's key to remain aware of the clutter we accumulate in our houses without even noticing and not to let it build up, to make sure that we're still in control of our spaces.

To do this, you will need to keep your problem areas in mind and constantly question whether how you are living – and what you're living with – is in line with your needs. Decluttering is a bit like cleaning your teeth – you need to keep on top of it every day. If you don't clean your teeth, plaque will build up and your teeth will fall out!

Likewise, if you don't keep on top of clutter, it can build up and you lose control. Consistency is key to maintaining your home.

You are the one person responsible for what comes into your home – and what keeps coming in.

Ready? Good! The first step to your decluttering journey is to start with a space audit...

HOW TO DO A SPACE AUDIT

Now that you've decided that you need to make a change, it's important to assess your space. You need to do a space audit. It's an extremely useful process, whether you're decluttering your own home or you're dealing with someone else's space (such as a parent's house). Sometimes, it can be hard to realise just how bad the situation is until you take a step back and try to look at it objectively. That is what a space audit aims to do.

STEP 1: ASSESS

Grab yourself a notebook and pen, walk out of your front door and lock it behind you. Take a few steps back (yes, even if you live in a flat) and look at where you live. Take it in and consider the value of the space behind your front door. Appreciate

that you have the keys to your own home, your own safe space and sanctuary, however messy it might have become. That's all that really matters. But in order to make your home amazing, in order for you to properly appreciate the space, you also need to be able to realise where you're going wrong, to work out what the problems are so that you can move on.

Now walk forwards very slowly, unlock the door and step inside. When you walk into your home, what are the first things that you see that you want to change?

Split your notebook page in two. On one side, write down what bothers you and why. What don't you like? What things are having an effect on you – emotionally or physically? What is there an excess of? What could you remove? What furniture doesn't work? On the other side, write down the things that you do like. What *does* work?

Take notes of everything you see and feel, answering all questions honestly.

Slowly walk through your home, taking in each room at a time and ask yourself the same questions.

How does each room make you feel when you walk into it? Does it feel inviting? Relaxing? Spacious? Or does it feel claustrophobic?

More often than not we just skim through life without stopping to really appreciate what we have or realising what the space we are currently living in is truly like. This exercise is meant to make you absorb your home slowly. Writing down all the issues you spot as you walk through your home will let you look at the space with fresh eyes and a greater attention to detail. This process is designed to clarify the areas that need the most attention.

STEP 2: PRIORITISE

Next, I would like you to think about what your ideal scenario would be. Imagine you could walk into each room and wave a magic wand and it would be just as you would like it. Write this dream description in your notebook.

Now is the time to plan how you can transform that vision into reality. Later in the book, I will guide you through how to do that, looking at how you can get that space to work. First, you need to work out what's stopping you from making that happen.

Write down a list of priorities for your home. If you want a place to congregate and eat Sunday lunch or a quiet space for the kids to do homework, add them to your list. Perhaps you want a multifunctional room for the kids to play in and do their arts and crafts, or you need a calm office area. Do you want a library or reading nook? Would you love to have an at-home fitness hub? Think about what is most valuable to the way you live *and* what each space would be most useful as.

STEP 3: VISUALISE

Think back to when you saw your home empty on moving day, before the boxes arrived. Or perhaps remember how your home looked the first time you saw it, when you walked round with the estate or letting agent. Try to recall the vision you had for your house or flat then.

If you don't have a vision, you're not going to know how to change the room and make it better.

Think about what you want that space to feel like. How do you want to feel when you're sitting down? What do you want within arm's reach? Are you watching TV or reading a book? Think about a memorable hotel room or your favourite space, then about how you can recreate even the tiniest part of that in your own house, with colours, texture, furniture, lighting or even scent.

How much do you want to change that space? Because if you really, really want to change it, you will. If you haven't got that vision, start looking at interior design accounts on Instagram. Build a Pinterest board. Subscribe to an interior design channel on YouTube. Watch

TV. These are times of financial hardship, so you don't have to pay anyone – there is free content and inspiration everywhere.

The most important thing at this stage is that you have to be *willing* to change. You need to *want* it.

I'm guessing that if you're reading this book, you've taken the first step.

STEP 4: RETHINK YOUR SPACE

If you were to take the plan of your home back to the drawing board, where might the best place for each item be? You can draw a floorplan and decide the positions on paper, but I suggest you play around with the furniture. What position allows the most light to flow into the room? Think practically – the furniture can't block any doors or windows – and remember that you always want to make sure that the maximum floor space is visible. Visible floor space is key because it gives the illusion of a bigger room. The more clutter and stuff that blocks your floor, the smaller the space looks, even if it's a large room.

Tip

Dilly's decluttering tips

1. Think about which space is most in need of change.

2. What is affecting your relationships or causing you the most stress?

3. Set aside time.

4. Write down a plan for what areas you need to tackle and in what order you are going to do it.

5. Do you need to buy any storage solutions?

6. Do you need to recruit another person to help?

7. Are you in the right place mentally to begin?

8. Can you dispose of what you need to declutter responsibly?

9. Research where your items can be distributed so you have a plan in place.

10. Just do it. Don't procrastinate, get started.

Think about what each specific room is used for. Does that room's purpose still make sense? Are there spaces that you can convert to use for another purpose that would suit your family better? Think about whether you can create zones in each room to dedicate to different activities.

It's extremely beneficial to realise that you don't need as much stuff as you think you did, too. If you have made a decision to get rid of some of your possessions, this will allow you to realise the value of the space around you. The space audit encourages you not to re-buy those items, because you can see that living in a clear space leaves you in a better mental state than being surrounded by clutter ever did.

If a room is full, we can't see its potential. If a room is empty, we can create a vision.

When you think of all your old possessions, you'll remember how much time you had to devote to tidying them and cleaning them – and the money you spent on them, too.

If you do need to replace something, follow the mantra of 'one in, one out'. This will ensure that you haven't cleared your space to simply add in more stuff again.

STEP 5: CLEAR YOUR SPACE

Throughout this book, I will encourage you to look at your space and constantly ask yourself how you might want to adapt it. To do this effectively, it is important to strip a room or cupboard back to an empty blank space before you can start to organise it. When I work on the BBC show *Sort Your Life Out* as a professional organiser, we empty the contents of every house into a warehouse. Taking your home back to a blank slate helps you to see things more clearly – it is the best way to work out how you can change it. If you can, empty each space out completely (moving the clutter and furniture into a garage, shed or spare room – or even the room next door, temporarily) and ask the most important question:

How can I make this room better?

Seasonal Planner

SPRING	SUMMER	AUTUMN	WINTER
Big Space 1: Entrance (see page 59)	Big Space 1: Garage/shed (see page 90)	Big Space 1: Bedroom/ wardrobes (see page 126)	Big Space 1: Kitchen (see page 158)
Dolly Dash 1: Mail (see page 61)	Dolly Dash 1: Paint store (see page 90)	Dolly Dash 1: Linen cupboard (see page 129)	Dolly Dash 1: Fridge/freezer (see page 159)
Big Space 2: Living room (see page 60)	Big Space 2: Utility room (see page 92)	Big Space 2: Loft (see page 130)	Big Space 2: Bathroom (see page 160)
Dolly Dash 2: Bookshelves (see page 64)	Dolly Dash 2: Cleaning supplies (see page 95)	Dolly Dash 2: Kids' things (see page 130)	Dolly Dash 2: Make-up bag (see page 161)

7-Day Challenge

SPRING	SUMMER	AUTUMN	WINTER
1 Let the light in – clear and clean windows *Remove 1 object from your space*	**1** Choose your capsule wardrobe *Remove 1 object from your space*	**1** Sweep chimneys *Remove 1 object from your space*	**1** Tackle your loungewear *Remove 1 object from your space*
2 Go through your bedlinen *Remove 2 objects*	**2** Clear out your handbag *Remove 2 objects*	**2** Toy tidy *Remove 2 objects*	**2** Clean appliance filters *Remove 2 objects*
3 Vacuum behind and under heavy items of furniture *Remove 3 objects*	**3** Clean windows inside and out *Remove 3 objects*	**3** Assess cooking equipment and clean oven *Remove 3 objects*	**3** Create a tea and coffee station; descale kettle *Remove 3 objects*
4 Clear and tidy the understairs or coat cupboard *Remove 4 objects*	**4** Refresh cushions, curtains and blinds *Remove 4 objects*	**4** Organise and recycle batteries *Remove 4 objects*	**4** Remove negative influences *Remove 4 objects*
5 Create a filing system for mail and paperwork *Remove 5 objects*	**5** Clean rugs and carpets *Remove 5 objects*	**5** Declutter arts, crafts and hobby items *Remove 5 objects*	**5** Clean mattresses *Remove 5 objects*
6 Tidy and clean your car interior *Remove 6 objects*	**6** Declutter chairs and stools *Remove 6 objects*	**6** Tidy magazines *Remove 6 objects*	**6** Refresh pillows *Remove 6 objects*
7 Unsubscribe from marketing emails *Remove 7 objects*	**7** Clean and assess suitcases and travel bags *Remove 7 objects*	**7** Clean gutters and sweep paths *Remove 7 objects*	**7** Declutter and tidy Christmas decorations *Remove 7 objects*

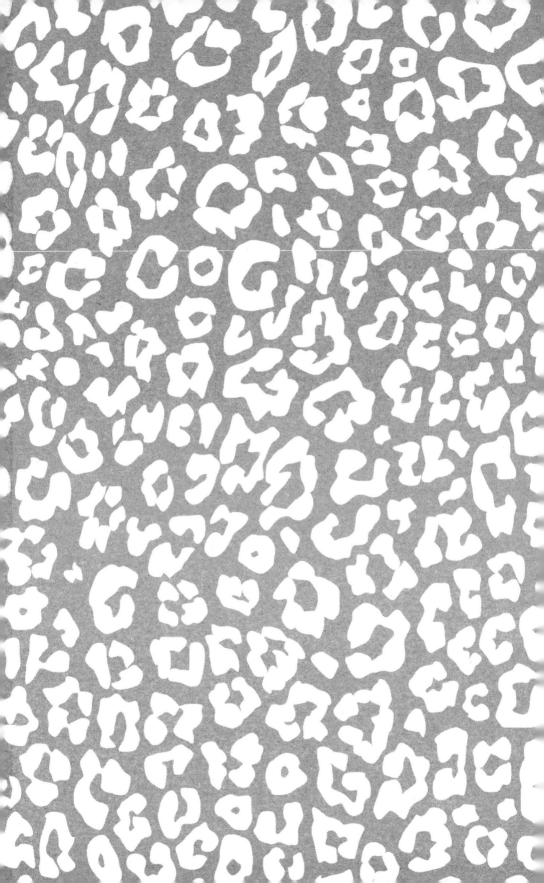

PART ONE

ADAPT

your space

ADAPT (verb), 1: to make (something) suitable for a new use or purpose; modify; **2:** to become adjusted to new conditions; to change your ideas or behaviour to make them suitable for a new situation.

MY STORY

It was never the plan for my mum to live with us. While it was clear she couldn't live alone, Charley and I certainly didn't have the money to send her to a residential home, and neither did she. My mum and dad, despite working every minute of the day, experienced a lot of financial difficulty. As newlyweds, Charley and I didn't have huge funds, so together with my mum we decided the most sensible option was to sell Mum's house and pool our resources to buy something together. Mum's mental health deterioration meant she needed constant care, so to keep an eye on her, the only option was to adapt a space to make it work for all of us.

Lots of people live in shared spaces, but in order to make it a success for us, we had to think hard and make a proper plan for how the situation could work. We found a house in the right location that had space at the bottom of the garden to build an annexe, but Mum would have to live with us until we could get the build done. For three years, she lived with us in our house, in our space, and it was tough!

While we were building the annexe, my mum had a tiny box bedroom upstairs. All it had in it was a bed and a rail of clothes. I felt constantly guilty that she was living in such a small space. Even though it had what she needed, I wanted to give her more. I couldn't give her any more space at the time, but because she was in our house, Mum was happy. She had the use of the main bathroom, as Charley and I are lucky enough to have an en suite, but downstairs was open-plan, so even something as basic as watching

TV became tricky. I soon realised that I needed to create an extra living area for Mum so she didn't encroach on our space and had a place that she could call her own too. The only option was to convert the conservatory, which we had been using as our daughter Nelly's playroom. We adapted it into Mum's living room, including a space for Jasmine the cat. (Not only did my mum move in with us, her cat came too! Did I mention Charley hates cats?)

First, we had to clear out Nelly's toys. Most went into her bedroom and we donated those she had outgrown. We emptied the rest of the space and brought in some furniture we had found locally. There was a sofa, coffee table and TV, but my main focus was that Mum had a comfortable space that was practical, too. We repurposed a trolley for her medicines and found an Ikea Kallax unit to organise all her books, photos and belongings, so she had everything she needed within arm's reach.

Throughout my life, my mum's illness has been a constant that I've learned to live with. But I've also learned how to adapt the space around us all to accommodate her needs and – equally importantly – allow her to have her own space. In those early days of living with us, Mum was at the height of her illness. Carers would come in three times a day, seven days a week, to look after her and make sure she was taking her tablets. Living with bipolar disorder and numerous other conditions means a huge amount of medication a day. However, I never minded this disruption because they would go straight to her part of the house. That physical separation stopped us feeling stressed about the constant comings and goings. The hardest part of living together was sharing a cooking space, but giving Mum her own living space changed everything.

She had relied very heavily on Charley and me to do most things for her. Interestingly, from the moment she moved into her own annexe, she became much more self-sufficient and her mental state improved. I realised that relying on us was debilitating her. By doing everything for her, we were – without knowing it – slowly de-skilling her and it was having a negative effect on her mental health. In the annexe, Mum was enjoying doing things for herself again.

This experience gave me first-hand knowledge of how having your own space (even if that is within a shared area) can be such a benefit to our mental health. Once people have control over their own space, be it one room, an area within a room or even a shelf, they feel more in control and things can improve. When we lose that control, we can struggle.

Organisation is a constant journey. It's not a one-stop shop.

When Mum moved into her own home, we changed the conservatory once more – this time into a multifunctional dining area – a place for Nelly to do her homework and for me to work from my laptop. When I'm not in someone's house, my workspace is at home (an experience I'm sure many of you are familiar with since WFH became the new normal). So, with the transition of my mum out of that space, we adapted it again to make an area that benefits us all.

Adapting is a constant in our lives. Clutter comes and goes, decreasing and increasing with life's journey, but it's important to stay aware of it, to stop things slipping backwards. My mum is in a much better place now, but I still need to help her stay tidy and organised. I have to go through her wardrobe regularly. I sort out the annexe kitchen cupboards and clear the fridge every week. Because Mum still suffers with her mental health, it's essential that she has that extra assistance.

It's a huge commitment to adapt your home and how you live in order to have other family members live with you. But it has had a really positive effect on me mentally. If you are helping someone that has helped you in the past, it feels like you're paying them back.

Try to always keep the positive reasons for why you're adapting your home at the front of your mind.

Finding space is not always easy. But if space is key to our wellbeing, then in order to carve some out in your home, be it a place for a parent, child or partner (or cat!), you need to be flexible, you need to be organised and you need to clear away the clutter that might be preventing you from finding that space.

KEY LIFE CHANGE

ADAPTING FAMILY SPACE

Multigenerational living is becoming more and more common. Due to economic pressures, young people are moving back home when they finish studying or aren't even moving out in the first place! It's not uncommon for younger couples to move in with their parents while they save towards or build their first home. More and more families are pooling their resources to buy homes where grown-up kids can keep an eye on elderly parents, while grandparents help out with childcare. (A dream – as much as it was lovely to think I might have 24/7 childcare when we moved in together, my mum couldn't look after my child – I was actually looking after Mum!)

If you have someone else living in your house, its really important to think about what will work best for all of you. There are some tough questions that you will need to ask yourselves and find the answers to when you're sharing a home. One of the first things to work out is how to give each person their own space. It could be a whole room or just a corner if you don't have that to spare. It might even be just a cupboard, or a shelf in the fridge, but everyone needs to have access to their own personal space to help them keep hold of their own identity and to give them some mental space, too. As you go through the process of adapting your space, it's really important that you add in clear physical boundaries by using furniture, storage, or even labels on boxes or drawers.

Clear boundaries will allow each person to know what space they have and it gives them a sense of control over their space too.

I'd like you to think about the rooms in your home. If you have a parent living with you, would it be better to sacrifice a playroom your child no longer uses or do you have a spare room you can convert into a living area? We all think about bathrooms and bedrooms as necessary private spaces, but everyone also needs a space of their own where they can watch TV, read a book, or do crafts or hobbies without intruding on others. If you're all sat on one sofa together, trying to watch one TV show, it can be difficult. So, give some serious thought to how you will carve out some space for each person somewhere in your home.

ZONING

When we moved into our house, there were three rooms downstairs, but we took out all the walls because we wanted open-plan living. We dreamed of having a huge extension,

tip

Timeshare

If you don't have physical space to spare, think about adapting the time you use certain rooms. Perhaps you let your parent have the front room on Monday and Tuesday nights so they can watch their favourite TV shows, while you go out for the evening. Drawing up a rota is always a good idea. Include all the activities that involve shared space. So, as well as TV time, add in cooking, laundry and bathroom time. When everybody in the house knows how you're sharing the space, it will give you all the opportunity to really be yourselves (whether that's trying new recipes in the kitchen or spending spa-time in the bathroom).

but because we had my mum living with us, we had to convert the conservatory into her living room instead. In lockdown, Charley built a wooden Scandi-style partition to split the open space, to separate our living, relaxing and functional areas. As much as we wanted to live open plan, it was important for us to give the living space a cosier feel for relaxing in – and divide that from the busy kitchen.

Partitioning is a really simple way to create different zones, whether that's for watching TV, eating or cooking. We found that adding a partition helps to divide up bigger spaces and allows our one large living area to feel like three different rooms. It has helped us to create an identity for each of those zones, as each space now serves a different purpose. You could do the same with your living/working/sleeping spaces to help you differentiate the areas. Partitions don't have to be physical walls but can also be pieces of furniture, such as a shelf divider, or a curtain.

In your house, think about what's going on and what zones *you* can create. Perhaps you might be thinking about a play area for kids or a relaxing area for adults. If all you need is a chair to cosy up in and read your book, think about whether there is a pocket of space in your hallway or on a landing that you can use for this. Perhaps you can think of outside space too... Another lockdown project saw Charley building a bar in our garden, which is an amazing social space.

tip

Look inwards before you look outwards

My house has always had an open-door policy. Ours is the social house, the party house. However, while I love to have friends over and want to look after them and give them the best time, it's important that you should never think about other people when you're buying a house or planning to adapt your own home.

Instead, be selfish. Thinking of others, when actually you should be thinking of yourself, is not helpful. Ask, what's most important to *me* or to *us*? What's most important to how you are living in this house, either on your own or as a family? Spare rooms for guests or bar areas are truly a luxury if you're struggling to live your daily lives in the space you have.

So many of us now are adapting our outside spaces to make new zones. You need to think: is there a way I can adapt my house to benefit my family or my lifestyle? It might seem like a large investment to buy an external shed or build a garden outhouse (or a bar!), but this could be the solution to living more calmly *in* your home if you really have run out of rooms.

WORKING FROM HOME

Since I wrote my first book, working from home has become the new normal. For many of us, our bedrooms or living rooms have become multitasking workspaces! Perhaps it's time for you to ask yourself if working from your bedroom or balancing your laptop on the sofa is really the best and most productive option. It's certainly unhealthy to sleep *and* work in your bedroom. The first thing you see when you wake up is your desk. Last thing at night? It's that desk. Likewise, bringing work into your family's leisure space is just as disruptive. You have a visible, constant reminder of work. It doesn't matter how much you might love your job, you still don't want to take it to bed with you or be thinking

about it in your downtime. You need to create some boundaries.

I recommend trying to separate your living and working spaces at home, so you can walk away from your work at the end of the day and transition back into home life. Differentiation is essential. Once you mix working and living spaces, it becomes very hard to separate them again. Finding a physical way to give closure to each day's work will help you function better and be more productive in the 'office'.

Compartmentalising your work, away from your living spaces, will stop you feeling that your personal space is being intruded on and allow you to properly relax.

When you work from home, how you adapt your space obviously depends on the job you have and the importance you place on your career. If your job is hugely important to you, I'd suggest that you prioritise creating an 'office' where no one else is going to interrupt you. If you don't physically define your work area, you'll find yourself in a stressful situation as you will likely be constantly interrupted by everything else going on in the house. Deciding how important a separate workspace is in your life will impact how you can think about changing your space. Once you have made this decision, the next step is deciding where you could create that environment.

FINDING SPACE

In order to create an effective workspace at home, you need to be able to switch into work mode and understand that that space equals work. When you walk out of your 'office' to make lunch in your kitchen, you're suddenly back in home mode. You might empty the dishwasher or put a load of washing on or pick up some of the kids' toys... If you're physically at work, you don't nip back home to do laundry in your lunch break, do you? I have found that even when you're working from home you need to avoid distractions for the whole day. When you're in a mixed space, you can't help but blend your work and home life together. Finding a physically different space is brilliant, if you can. Ideally, you need a room that you can walk into and close the door, like a real office. Consider whether you have space in your garden to build a garden office

or adapt a shed or outbuilding into a WFH room. Make sure there is a coffee machine and a fridge in that space and you will be able to work a full day without being distracted by your house or home life.

If you're looking to find an office space inside your home, look at whether you can prioritise the rooms differently. If your kids have a playroom, could that be converted into an office space? You need to weigh up what would be more beneficial to you and the way you live in your home. Perhaps your child is older and only uses the playroom for an hour after school, or maybe they prefer to play in their bedroom. Even if they use it semi-regularly, if you're working for eight hours a day in a cramped corner, it makes more sense to convert that playroom into an office.

Is there a spare room or do you have a space under the stairs? Could you add a desk into a corner of your living room? I want to encourage you to think deeply about adapting the space you have, depending on your changing priorities.

Try to avoid creating a workspace in the bedroom. Your bedroom should always be a relaxing space, a calm sanctuary.

If you are lucky enough to have a spare room, ask yourself how often you actually have guests over to stay. Maybe every six months? Once a year at Christmas? If you got rid of the bed and moved in a desk, you've got yourself an office! If someone really needs to stay with you, they could sleep on the sofa (or you could get a sofa bed). Remember that *you* live in your house 365 days of the year, while your guest is only there for one night. No one really needs a spare room, but we *do* need all our rooms to have a clearly defined purpose, which will make living in your house an easier experience.

WHEN MORE THAN ONE PERSON WORKS FROM HOME

If you live with someone who also works from home, you might find yourselves arguing about whose job is more important and who deserves a dedicated space to work in. Perhaps your WFH arrangements are affecting your relationship.

Maybe you are stuck at the kitchen table, when there's a bigger room dedicated to something else that's only used for a couple of hours a week. Decide what's most important to you and work out how the situation makes you feel.

It's always going to be a problem working out who gets to take priority over a working area if you share your home. A good place to start is for both of you to write down the top three things you need to do your job. Consider these points (warning: there could be arguements!):

1. Whose career is more important to them? Or are they of equal importance?

2. Are you spending most of the day on calls?

3. Do you need privacy?

4. Who needs the most space (whether that's space to carry out tasks for your job or space to store files and materials)?

5. Who needs a good Zoom background?

6. Do you need good lighting?

When you each have your top three needs, it's up to you to calmly work it out and decide which space in your house will tick each of your requirements. You definitely need to think about adapting and sharing the space you have *equally*. If you rotate the furniture, maybe you could both work in one room together. If not, how about rotating your time instead? One of you could use the home office for half the week, the other has it the remaining days. Alternatively, you could split it by morning and afternoon. You could each work from the kitchen for half the time, then switch, depending on what you're doing. Adapting your schedules or working spaces to really work for you both can help to ensure you are happier in your home.

CHANGING ROOMS

It's time to weigh up the value of each room.

For each room in your home, write down a list of priorities that address everyone in the family's needs, in terms of time and space, and make a plan:

1. Who needs to spend time in that room?

2. What happens in the space?

3. Is the furniture enhancing or overwhelming the space? Is it too big? Is there too much of something?

4. What is stopping the room from functioning as it needs to?

5. Can the furniture be moved to make the space work better?

6. What is in the room that doesn't naturally belong there? What can you reduce and remove to enhance the space in the room?

It's a good idea to frequently ask yourself: how is your space and the stuff in it affecting the relationships in your household and the way people are living? For example, if you have children and their toys are strewn everywhere, but at the same time your spare room is full of clothes you never wear, it's time to reassess how you are using your rooms.

When I help clients who are moving house, I see so many parents choose the biggest bedroom for themselves, then never reevaluate that choice. But further down the line you might find you need to switch rooms and adapt the way you are living. If you have a child, you may have given your baby the smallest room when they were born, but now they're bigger does it make more sense to give them the largest bedroom? If they're sociable, they can hang out in their room with their friends, rather than taking over the living room! If you have teenagers, they might benefit from having a bedroom with an ensuite, or perhaps you can switch them to a smaller room if they have gone off to university and only come back from time to time.

As you evolve as a family, even without anyone else moving in, it's important to constantly look at the bedrooms and bathrooms in your home, to ensure you're still using the space effectively.

Do a deep dive to find out what is key to your mental wellbeing. Perhaps you need a gym at home because you love to exercise. Maybe you'd rather go into the office or work in a shared space than lose a space that houses your home fitness kit. Or maybe you're willing to sacrifice an office space because your kids really need a playroom.

Constantly re-assess your priorities and, if you need to, make a change.

KEY QUESTIONS ON SPACE SHARING

1. Is everyone living in the most practical room or space for their stage in life?

2. Could you prioritise the rooms in your home differently?

3. Can you create zones to mark out different areas?

4. Could you consider time-sharing spaces?

THE BIG PICTURE

A lot of people may say, 'Oh, I'm a bit of a hoarder,' but there is a huge difference between someone that buys in excess and likes to keep hold of their belongings and a person that has been diagnosed with hoarding disorder (which was recognised as a distinct mental illness in 2013). Symptoms include: an inability to get rid of your things and extreme levels of stress when you try to throw things out; anxiety about needing things in the future (which is different to keeping hold of things 'just in case'); uncertainty about where to put your things; being distrustful about other people touching your belongings; and rooms becoming so full of stuff you can't actually use them or even open the doors because they are blocked with clutter. It's more prevalent in the elderly and can be treated with medical assistance. Most of the homes that I deal with, however, are not real hoarder's houses. If you feel close to being overwhelmed by your clutter, you may not have a medical disorder, you have probably just got too many things. But if you've reached that point, it's definitely time to break old patterns and embed new, positive behaviours that will change your relationship with your possessions.

THE SPENDING CYCLE

What I see so often is that someone's love for shopping or the buzz that they get from buying a new top each week tends to spiral into a situation where it becomes two tops a week, and then something new every day. Before they know it, there is a stack of packages by the front door that haven't even been

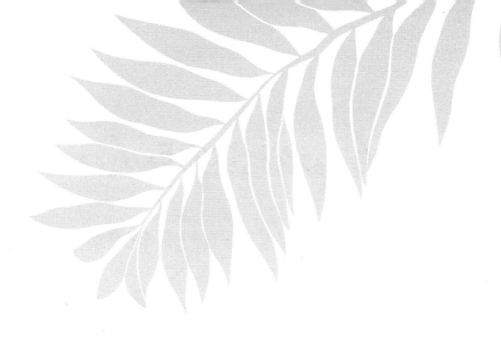

opened, because there are so many. They have no idea what they've bought – or what they already own. It's clear that they've reached a point where their spending habits are out of control. I'm using the example of clothes, but really it could be anything bought in excess: books, mugs, ornaments, tinned foods...

We consume for so many different reasons other than to satisfy our basic needs. I've seen people who use shopping as a way to fill a void. The thrill of pressing the 'buy now' button is exciting – an instant high to dissipate their feelings of depression or anxiety for a short while. I've also witnessed plenty of clients who are swayed into thinking that they've got a good deal because an item is on sale. But if the tags are never taken off, it's not a bargain.

Often people think about things that they don't have and want to buy them to fill that gap... but I think it's always essential to bring it back to the basic questions:

Have I got space for it?

Do I really need it?

Ask yourself, where does this behaviour stem from?

And if it's damaging, how can I try to break that cycle?

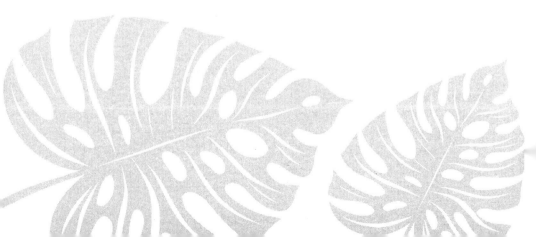

BREAKING THE CYCLE

Physical clutter is often a result of our mental state, and how we consume often reflects how our parents shopped and shaped our upbringing. For people that have come from very little or started with nothing, I've seen them over-compensate. As soon as they feel they've got some spare money in their pockets, they will buy. Then they buy some more. And more. It's a very common trait I've seen in many of the homes I've worked in. The thinking is often that they once had nothing and as they can now afford the clothes/shoes/handbags, they will buy them *just because they can*. Similarly, parents who had few toys when they were children make a choice to buy everything their child wants. So much of the 'decluttering' process is actually about deciphering your own thought-processes around your belongings and how you approach accumulating them.

For those who recognise these scenarios, it's essential to look back at what you had during childhood and what you have now to see the correlation. You need to break that cycle and not cling to a behaviour that is influenced by your past. Just because you didn't have any toys then, that doesn't mean you child has to be spoiled now. Yes, you want to make sure that your kid has good things in their life, but they still need to learn to appreciate everything they are given and to also appreciate the value of their toys. I have seen families who buy 300+ toys for each child at Christmas. My husband Charley is exactly the same. He also feels that our daughter has to have hundreds of presents under the tree. His thinking is that children love to open presents, so why not give her more? But why are we giving so much to our children? I'd like you to keep asking yourself, how did I get to be like this? Where does this behaviour stem from? Did I inherit it or learn it? And if it's unhelpful, how can I try to break that cycle?

We learn a lot of amazing things from our parents, but when you are a parent yourself, you need to be very careful about what you show your kids. The more negative you are about your space, the more that negative energy will feed into everyone else in the house. I recommend that you always try to create positive spaces for the whole family. Children pick up on what's around them very quickly and they learn by what they see. Whether it's your attitude to your home, or the fact that you're constantly shopping, or whether you always make your bed in the morning, children see those actions and take those learned behaviours into their own lives. How you live now could cause negative behaviours in the years to come, whether that's spending too much or living with clutter. Consider what your children see you doing day in, day out. They can't help but absorb what we are teaching them.

Educate your children to ensure they become organised – it's a skill for life. If your teenager loves fashion, teach them not to buy from cheap fast-fashion retailers and to ignore the influencers telling them to buy clothing that costs just £5. Guide them away from fast fashion or they could end up filling the home with too many poor-quality clothes that are worn once and then end up in a landfill. My daughter Nelly-Reet is currently eight years old. She has a very small wardrobe and three drawers. I don't buy her more clothes unless she goes through her stuff and gets rid of things she's grown out of, doesn't wear or doesn't need. She doesn't see me buying new things all the time so she's learning through my example. I do buy occasional good-quality items, but there's not a new package of throw-away fashion coming into the house every week.

CREATE A SPENDING LOG

Perhaps it's time to own up to how many Amazon deliveries you're getting a day. When you looked at your bank statement from last month, how much did you spend on clothes? And how much did you spend on going out for coffees or lunches? If you spend £50 a week at Primark as a distraction activity, because you're bored in your lunch break, think about how else you could spend that money.

If you have no idea where your money goes, it's a very eye-opening exercise to create a spending log. Make some time to sit down with your bank and credit card statements and add up what you are spending on different items each month. Make columns for bills and other essential household expenses, such as your rent, mortgage and insurance. Make a column for supermarket and grocery shops. Then make columns for clothing, eating out, coffee-shop visits and little luxuries. If there's something you know you buy in excess, put it on the list and work out how much you are spending on it each week or month. A picture will begin to emerge...

Channel the money you've been spending mindlessly on things you don't need into creating a better living environment for yourself or your family. You will have to sacrifice some things, but always work out what you think is worth it. I don't have time to clean my house, so I would rather have someone clean it for me and buy fewer clothes. Work out what is more valuable to you and what is better for your mental health. If you pay someone to do two hours of cleaning with the savings you've made from not buying fast fashion, you get back two hours of time to focus on something that *is* important to you. You could probably afford a cleaner, someone to do your ironing or a person who could organise your house once a week. You're *choosing* not to. You're *choosing* to waste that money on shoddy clothes and takeaway coffee.

If you really want to make a change, to adapt that space, to get in control of your house, it's only *you* who can break the habit and you need to ask yourself the following:

1. How long have you been feeling like this?

2. Have you asked for help before?

3. Has anyone offered to help you?

4. Have you ever tried to declutter before?

5. Can you improve your situation yourself?

6. Could your family get involved?

7. Is it a case for external help?

Once you've realised you need to make a change, reach out and ask for help – whether that's from your friends, family, a professional organiser or even a team of declutterers.

If you really want to make a change, to get in control of your house, it's only YOU who can break the habit.

47

LOOK AFTER YOURSELF

How you feel in your house is more important than anything else.

We very quickly become attached to bricks and mortar, but it is just a house and you can recreate your home anywhere. How you function in that space relates to how the space affects you – how it makes you feel. Some people are miserable in their own houses and it can be because they don't know how to effectively adapt their space. I think it's time to ask: do you love the situation you're in? If you don't, how can you change it? Try to work out if you can make your house more multifunctional and consider what you could do better. If you're reading this book, I'm guessing you've already come to the point where you know things need to change. I talk about it constantly,

but if you want to create change, you have to be ready to do the work.

And get ready to welcome all the wellbeing benefits – the calmness, the sense of achievement – that will come when you've done it. So, what we have to ask is this: is it the house, the contents or the people that are the issue? Write down a list with separate sections for the problems with your house, the issues you face living there and the problems you have around the clutter in your home.

> If you need a utility room, that would be in the house section.

> If someone new is coming to live in your house, that would be a living issue.

> If you have too many shoes in your wardrobe and you can't see what you own any more, that is a problem with clutter.

For each problem there will be a solution, but you will often have to make a sacrifice for it to work, whether that's having two children share a room or giving up a study for a parent to stay. Only you can decide whether you need to change the space, or to change what's *in* the space. People are quick to exclaim that they need another room, but often it isn't the space that is the problem, it's the amount of clutter in that space.

Only you can decide whether you need to change the space, or to change what's in the space.

Think about it: the reason we often take our laptops and sit in coffee shops when we WFH is because we don't want to be at home. We leave our house to work because we want to be more productive. We go into the office because we know we're going to be able to focus. But I'd like you to think about the fact that you should *want* to be in your space,

rather than escape it. I see so many people who just don't want to be in their houses. They feel their space is too stressful to work in, so they are forced to go elsewhere. For a lot of people, the mess in their house actually makes them miserable. If that feels like the situation you're in, you can change this.

Every time you go round your house and think about what you could improve, go out the front door and follow the process of the space audit on page 20. Always be grateful for the fact you have a roof over your head. Once you've figured out what you need your space to be, and when it's working for you, your home life will start to flow perfectly. You'll be amazed at the difference it can make to your life. A calm and organised home or workspace will help you to focus on the tasks at hand. A calmer space = more productivity.

COST CONSIDERATIONS
– MOVE OR IMPROVE?

If you want to adapt a room, write down the three main issues within your home that you feel you're living with right now. Are the people in your home unhappy? Are your relationships strained? Is it that you feel there isn't enough space? Does it feel like you're drowning in stuff? Or is the issue that you have more people in the house than before? Assess what is causing the problem. Often, it's the sheer excess of what you own. But beyond decluttering, is there anything else you can do?

As an example, if I was to have another baby right now, and we couldn't afford to move to a home with another bedroom and an annexe for my mum, we would have to turn the spare room into a nursery. It's currently used as a walk-in wardrobe, so the clothes would have to move to our bedroom, which would make it smaller. We don't have many clothes, but we've still got too many for that space. So we would have to ask ourselves: what is going to be the best financial expenditure that will benefit the whole of our family? For us, I see the main options as being: 1) moving house; 2) building an extension or converting the space; or 3) reducing the amount of clothing we own. We would have to work out what would be more beneficial to us as a family. What are the options in your situation? That's what I'd like you to think about.

If you're in a financial position to do so, you might think about adding an extension to your house or doing a loft conversion. If so, you need to consider whether it will make your house more valuable in the long run. Every street has a ceiling price, so you need to keep in mind what is worth doing and why.

Whenever I make structural improvements, I constantly think: 'What if we sell this house?'

However, it's equally important not to get too swayed about what an estate agent might say a couple of years down the line. As well as keeping an eye on the long term, you need to focus on what's happening in your house RIGHT NOW. You might lose money in the future, but in the present moment, this feels really important. So what is more valuable to you? You can't predict what's going to happen in the future, so make the right decisions regarding what's going to improve your life right now.

If you're not in the position to make drastic and (let's face it) expensive changes, there are other ways to change your space. Start by looking at the space you have and work out how you can make rooms within rooms.

Consider how you can create identity for the people living within each space. Assess each room and list what you need to do to make it better. Write down what you can reduce and what you need to bring in to make the room work better for you all right now. Decluttering will always help you see a clearer way of how you can live in your space.

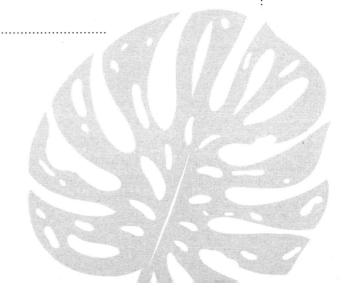

TIDY TIPS

Think back to student living or your first flat-share... I'll bet you became very territorial about your space, whether it was a cupboard in the kitchen or a shelf in the bathroom. What is more important than ever, when you're living in a shared space, is that you are in control of what you have in that space and that your space isn't overruling anyone else's. You have to be really, really minimal and in control of what you've got. When you come to live with other people, you have to give each other equal space, so that there are no arguments.

Even if you move into a more intimate situation, such as moving in with a partner, the same rules apply. For instance, if you have more clothes and your partner is happy for you to take over the majority of the storage options, that's fine. But you should still try to limit yourself. If you and your partner have a wardrobe each, and theirs is only half full, I would still encourage you to intentionally shop as though you have just one wardrobe. Likewise, if you've got a huge amount of clothes that are spilling into the spare room, it's going to create problems when someone stays over. What happens when you need to get your clothes out of the wardrobe, but you've got a guest? You're intruding on someone else's space.

The problems begin when we start to fill space that isn't ours.

When you are in shared living spaces, you always have to think about how much of your ego is represented by physical stuff. Is the stuff that I own in *my* space? Or is it spreading into someone else's space? If you have a bathroom with three shelves, shared between three people, make sure that you only take one shelf. We all have too much stuff already, and so often I work with people who think their only issue is decluttering and tidying when they then realised they were inadvertently taking over their partner's space.

REDUCE, DON'T FILL SPACE

If you move and are lucky enough to gain a spare room, it's tempting to think that you have 'free' space, so you keep buying things to fill it. But the more space you take over with your belongings, the more stressful life becomes, because you will still have to keep cleaning it and tidying it.

In every area of your home, it's important to constantly go through your belongings, decluttering, and working out what you don't need. Seeing your possessions clearly is essential, because if you don't know what you already have, you're just going to add to it, until suddenly your stuff has taken over someone else's space.

A good rule to follow is to only buy something if you're replacing an older item.

Live by the mantra of: one in, one out.

If you're planning to move in with someone else, I'd advise you to think carefully about what you take with you. Or, if someone is making the big move into *your* home (for example, your parents are coming to live with you), I suggest that you work out together what they are going to bring with them. How much do they really need?

A lot of the time we put belongings into storage and only just bring the basics into a new home. But ask yourself: why you are using a storage unit to store things you don't need for months on end? Storage is expensive, so before you consider it, ask yourself what you're keeping and why. Is it really worth it?

Letting go of things you never use is an incredibly energising and freeing process.

CREATING A MULTIFUNCTIONAL SMALL SPACE

Successfully living in a small space relies on only bringing the bare minimum into that space.

Four sets of cutlery and crockery is more than enough if living alone or with a partner. A multifunctional table that you can use for eating and working is essential. You'll only need two sets of bed linen and two sets of towels (one to be used while the other is in the wash) and I would recommend under-bed storage to house all the things you don't need to use every day. An ottoman that does double duty as a coffee table and opens up to provide storage will also be useful, so keep an eye out for furniture with hidden storage.

Never bulk-buy, whether that's groceries or cleaning products. Consider utilising wall space. Look up and add wall hooks, cupboards or shelving closer to the ceiling to create more space.

The other essential process when you're living in a small space is to deal with everything immediately, particularly post, parcels or piles of items to donate or that are for recycling. Otherwise, things will pile up fast and it's easier to get overwhelmed far more quickly in smaller spaces.

ZONING SOLUTIONS

Whether you're in a studio or a larger living space, dividing a room to create smaller zones is a great way to use it for multiple purposes. Open-backed bookshelves are great pieces of furniture if you want to create a divide – they're not a solid item that will block out precious light. Ikea's Kallax unit, glass bookshelves, open shelves that stand alone... all these can create a small divide within your space. You will find that a physical divide will also give you mental space too.

HEADING TO UNI OR MOVING IN WITH FRIENDS

If you're heading off to university or moving into a shared flat/house for the first time, try to buy a storage bed or at least have a selection of storage containers neatly stacked under your bed to keep your space tidy.

Get yourself a slim, tall cupboard or chest of drawers (often called a tallboy) that you can slot into a shared bathroom to put all your products in. If there isn't room, use a crate or box, so that instead of having your belongings spread across shelves, you know your things are in *your* container.

It completely depends on how many people are sharing the kitchen, but if you do have a drawer to yourself, split it into sections for cutlery, utensils and tea towels. I like to use drawer dividers to keep things neat, then label each section. You can also make sections for your crockery and glasses. With the cupboards or shelves, divide – and label – your items so you have sections for tins, dry goods and packets (like pasta) and cereals. Get some containers to decant things into or even a large Tupperware to house all your fridge items. If there isn't room for cupboard space, or even a shelf, you could get yourself a trolley that you keep in your room and wheel in, when necessary.

RETURNING FROM UNI OR MOVING BACK IN WITH PARENTS

When an adult child moves back into the family home, an adaptation of the living space is usually necessary. Ask yourselves, 'What is the most effective way we can exist in this space without affecting each other?' Is there an option for them to have a bedroom with an ensuite? Or can they have the bedroom closest to the bathroom? It's time to plan how it's going to work with minimal disruption. And, of course, you also want to make sure that they retain as much of their own identity and space as possible. Could you put a fridge in their room? Can you bring in a trolley for their bathroom items to keep them from cluttering up a shared space?

Always think about how you can make the space as comfortable for them as it is for you.

This is also the perfect opportunity to create a rota, so you can share the time in any multi-purpose spaces and think about zoning here, too.

WORKING FROM HOME

Whatever your job is, I think it's very important to make sure that the space immediately surrounding your WFH area feels accepting of your work. Maybe that means you have relevant books or files full of papers on shelves behind your desk. Even if your workspace is the end of your kitchen table, you need to feel like you are in a work zone.

If you can't carve out a dedicated workspace (see the tips on page 52), a trolley is a brilliant way to create a flexible working area. If you need to move to a quieter space, you can put your laptop, textbooks, or any paperwork on there and move from one room to another without it affecting anyone. At the end of the day, you can also wheel that trolley under the stairs or shut it in a cupboard so you don't have to look at it until the next day.

NEXT STEPS: REFINING

Once the space is working for everybody, I'd encourage you to ask the question: is it lovely? Your parents are sitting in the conservatory and they've got their own TV, but is it comfortable enough for them? You may have started off with a pretty basic spare room, with only just space for a bed, so to move to the next level, think about transforming that space into something really special.

It's so empowering when you see the benefits of adapting your home. In the first place, you're going to feel amazing because you've looked after the people that mean the most to you, but there are other positives, too. Knowing that your loved ones are safe and comfortable, that their needs are met; or having a dedicated workspace, where you can shut yourself away without the worry that someone else might need to use the room; or eradicating the dread of waking up every morning and seeing your work in front of you, will have immense benefits to your entire wellbeing.

SEASONAL PLANNER
Spring

Spring is naturally the time of adapting; it's the season of change, a time for new shoots, for shedding heavy winter layers and preparing the ground for a new start. It's the perfect time to have a good clear-out.

The seasons really affect us and how we live in our homes. Winter makes me want to hibernate, stay in, get blankets and cosy up on the sofa, but when spring arrives I want everything fresh and clean.

So, open the doors, open the windows, let the light in.

Spring gives everyone the chance for a fresh start and the opportunity to let go of everything. I'd like you to make the most of the season and ensure that you *are* letting go and readying yourself for a huge declutter.

You could start every season by following my 30 Days of Change Challenge (see page 167 for details of how to get stuck in) to completely refresh your space, but if you have less time to spare, start with the 7-Day Challenge (see page 178) or simply focus in on a key area instead.

In this section, I'm going to give you tips for sorting out two big areas: the entranceway and the living room. Choose one (or both!) and then pick two smaller areas that you could Dolly Dash.

Make your entrance a calm and pleasurable space to walk into.

BIG SPACE 1: ENTRANCE

Spring is a great time to make your entry space, whether it is a porch or hallway or even just the area immediately next to the door, a real *entrance*. Let that hopeful feeling of spring encourage you to create a fresh and welcoming entry space. This place is the very first thing you see when you open your front door – so make it a calm and pleasurable space to walk into.

I'll admit, my entrance is often a dumping ground. There are always different deliveries for when I'm creating content, but if you don't take care of packages as soon as they arrive, the area can very quickly become chaotic. It's easy to become blind to the things in our house that we need to work on, particularly at the front door. You walk in and out that door so many times that it's likely you will ignore everything about the space, because you're either rushing to get somewhere, or so relieved to be home. But it's the first place that visitors see, so it's a great place to get started. Make sure that the only items you have in that space are ones that need to be there and follow these steps...

1. CLEAR
Empty out everything from the area.

2. ORGANISE
Group all the items you've removed into sections:

> Coats

> Hats

> Gloves

> Scarves

> Dog leads and accessories

> Shopping bags

> Shoes

> Boots

> Sports equipment

3. RATIONALISE
Go through each of those sections and repair, donate or recycle hats that have holes in them or gloves your kids have outgrown. Does every glove have its pair? Does everyone still wear or use everything? Get rid of any items that don't get used.

4. CREATE STORAGE

Make sure that you have enough storage to cover all the people in your house and the different types of items that you need in this area of your home.

> A set of narrow tall drawers (a tallboy) could house the hats, gloves, scarves, dog equipment and shopping bags, with a dedicated drawer for each item.

> Create a shelf for shoes or add a basket to keep them tidy and in one place. A great idea for families is to create a dedicated shoe basket for each person – no more searching through a jumbled pile for shoes that match every morning!

> Do you have room for a storage bench, one that sits neatly in your hallway and that can store shoes and keep hats and gloves tucked away?

> Could you fit in a slimline wall-mounted storage cabinet?

> Attach some hooks or a rack for your coats to the wall. Ensure each member of your family has at least one hook.

> Create a dedicated box for mail.

5. MAKEOVER EXISTING STORAGE

If you have a hall or under-stairs cupboard, is it full of things you rarely use or items stacked on top of one another? Clear it out and think about whether you could add shelves and fill them with storage boxes for each group of items. Could you add coat hooks inside to keep winter coats out of the way while you are using summer ones? Wall-mounted racks can help keep sports equipment accessible and neat.

BIG SPACE 2: LIVING ROOM

1. PLAN

First ask: Is this room working the way you want it to? Is the layout the best? I suggest that you always begin by looking at the layout of the room. Imagine the room as an empty space and think about what you could do differently. Work out if the sofa is in the best place, the side tables, the bookshelves, the TV...

To do this, it's a good idea to draw the room plan out to scale on a piece of paper. Measure your items of furniture and draw them to scale too on separate bits of paper, then cut them out. You're then able to

Mail

One tiny thing that will make a huge impact is actually opening the mail when it arrives. Mail is a real struggle for a lot of people because it is often negative and it physically comes through your door into your house. A lot of the time letters are asking for something – bills, demands, commitments. That's why you put off opening them. They're either going to ask you to do something or ask for money. I only get fun mail once a year on my birthday!

When you do open those letters, you'll find that most of it isn't relevant or doesn't really matter. You've been putting off a task that was really easy to tackle and will make a huge difference to your entryway.

Even if it's junk mail, get into the habit of opening it, then returning to sender or recycling it.

Remove yourself from the mailing lists of catalogues you bought something from just once or brochures from brands you no longer shop with.

A digital detox is just as important. Go through your email inbox and unsubscribe from all the marketing mailers you're receiving. Brands want you to buy from them, but you know that you shouldn't be bringing any more stuff into your house, nor do you want to be spending money all day long. If you don't unsubscribe, you're going to keep getting constant reminders. Stop them.

move them around your room plan until it flows the way you'd like it to. Remember to look at the layout with the big-ticket furniture items, before you look at the smaller things.

2. CLEAR AND REARRANGE

In order to physically rearrange a room, you need to take out the smaller items first, before you move the larger items. Clear all the surfaces. I always recommend that you actually *remove* the items, instead of just trying to visualise the room differently, as it will give you the clearest view of how to move forward. We get so used to seeing things in one position, we can become blind to any other options. Sometimes it's hard to take sofas and sideboards out of a room, but if you take out all the other smaller items, it'll give you the space to move the bigger things around, to play with the layout. Making these physical changes will help you understand how the room might look better and flow more smoothly.

Of course, you might move it all around and decide it worked best how you had it in the first place! But at least you've tried. You now definitely know that this is the only configuration of furniture that will work for you.

3. DECLUTTER

Once you have settled on the layout, look inside any cupboards and on shelves. What are you housing? Books? Games? Kit for old hobbies? Random things you don't actually use any more? What could those shelves or cupboards be better used for?

As we move through life we are constantly evolving. Our jobs, careers and priorities change. Children grow up, our tastes change, technology changes. Different people come in and out of your life. It's key to adapt your home to how you live now. As children get older, we might decide to keep classic board games but get rid of all the ones that they don't play with any more. You might have shelves of DVDs but now you just watch Netflix. Are you still pursuing the hobbies that interested you years ago?

Always ask, what's working for you as a family right now?

As a rough guide, these are things that might be considered bare essentials for your living room:

> Sofa

> TV

> Side tables

> Console or sideboard or bookshelf

> Music system

> A few ornaments and books

And these are items that *don't* need to be there:

> Washing piles

> Ironing board

> Office work or kids' homework or schoolbooks

> Kids' toys

SOLUTIONS TO COMMON LIVING ROOM PROBLEMS

> Books – rationalise to a minimum, then organise neatly by genre

> CDs – get rid!

> DVDs – get rid!

> Vinyl – arrange attractively

> Ornaments – rationalise to a minimum then display beautifully

> Toys and games – only keep the ones that get used and find a neat and attractive storage solution for them that keeps them out of your eyeline

> Hobby equipment – keep what you use and store away effectively

> Unhung pictures or an excess of photo frames – moving them onto the wall could free up space

> Paperwork – file in purpose-made folders and boxes, and move to a dedicated office area

> Magazines, newspapers and brochures – get rid or organise collections neatly

> Clothes – laundry piles are often dumped in living rooms – iron them, if needed, straight away and store the clothes where they belong in the bedrooms

Bookshelves

Books can be hard to declutter, but it does depend on what type of reader you are. Some people read a book and don't feel they need it any more. Others keep every single book they have ever read. If you're not naturally the type to read it once and pass it on, you need to get brutal. You might love the idea of having a collection of books because they're classics, or because you plan to pass them down, or DEFINITELY read again... But stockpiling books and never going through them is a problem.

There's a Japanese word, *tsundoku*, which means buying books with the intention of reading them but never getting round to it. Ask yourself if you are actually going to read each book. Then consider if anyone else in the house will read them. If it's a no, they have to go.

I've found that books make up a huge percentage of the things we own that we don't actually need. We're rarely going to pass them on as heirlooms, so if someone else can have them *and* benefit, that's great. Ask your local libraries and schools if they need donations. If you have a stack of cookbooks you rarely use, you might decide that you don't need the physical books any more. So many recipes are online now. The only cookbook that I have – and use – is a Sri Lankan one that my mum found for me. I would never get rid of that book and I'll pass it down to Nelly too. These books of great sentimental importance are definitely ones you should keep. Book collections are lovely as long as they don't overwhelm the rest of your space.

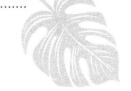

WELLBEING BENEFITS

When you've created space for somebody...
When you've given your parents their home back...
When you've created an office for your partner to work from instead of being cramped over the kitchen table...
When you've given your kids a playroom and you can see that they are playing more creatively...
When you're no longer looking at piles of paperwork in your bedroom...
When you've reduced the rails of clothes in your spare room, and created a reading nook...

1. Everyone will feel energised by the calmness of the spaces.

2. You will see the positive effect it has on your personal relationships, not just with yourself, but with the other people in your home.

3. You'll see the results of how important adapting your home is for everybody and you'll know it's been worth it because everyone is living in harmony.

4. A tidy, clutter-free house and workspace will improve your focus and help establish good working patterns.

LIFE LESSON

Realising that you need to adapt your home is a big commitment. I understand just how much it takes to acknowledge the change that is required, as I'm living through it with my own mum and I have seen it with families I've worked with time and again. But it can be hard.

Just because something belongs to you, doesn't mean you should keep it for the rest of your life.

Adapting can take many forms. One woman I worked with had so many clothes, they were spread out across every bedroom in the house. Her children's wardrobes didn't house their own clothes – they had her clothes in them! We got rid of so much together, although it was tough. She didn't want to give up anything. At the end of the process, we still had too much to store in her own wardrobes, so the solution was to rotate her wardrobe seasonally and keep half of it in the loft. And the children got their wardrobes back!

If you are someone that loves fashion but you have so many pieces that they are taking over your kids' bedrooms, it's time to admit that you have an obsession you can't control. If you are making your kids share a room so you can use a bedroom as a dressing room, *you* are the problem! You have to face facts that you are shopping uncontrollably to the detriment of your entire family and your children.

Up until the point I arrived, that family had learned to live in a pattern of misery. So perhaps you need to ask yourself whether you are living in a similarly repetitive cycle that is never going to change.

It can have a huge impact on your relationships, good and bad, but in order to change, sometimes difficult decisions need to be made.

Your home is a living space, not a storage space.

Another family I worked with had a large garage that needed to be converted so their grandparents could move in with them. A problem I see time and time again is that garages can encourage you to keep and store excess belongings. If you're not using it to park a car, think about how you could adapt the space to improve your lives, instead of just using it as a storage container. A garage could be your new office or a gym.

Follow this family's example and ask, what do I need this space for the most? This family really took hold of that idea and acted on it. They made an amazing decision to adapt their home that changed all their lives for the better.

PART TWO

SHARE

your space

SHARE (noun), 1: a part or portion
of a larger amount or item, which is
divided among a number of people,
or to which a number of people
contribute; (verb); **2:** to give a portion
of (something) to another or others;
3: use, occupy, or enjoy (something)
jointly with another or others.

MY STORY

I spent the first three years of my life in an orphanage in Sri Lanka. The first time my adoptive parents saw me was in a photo that one of their friends, the local bishop, had shown them. He knew they were looking to adopt a baby. I was only seven weeks old. The adoption process was hugely different in the early 1980s, so by the time my parents finally took me home it was 1983. I'm not really sure why it took that long, but by that point I was the oldest child in the orphanage.

The orphanage was bare and stark. The walls were made of stone and completely empty of paintings or drawings. There was no colour, no softness at all and there certainly weren't many toys. Actually, there wasn't much of anything, but whatever there was was shared. I didn't know any other way. From my earliest days, I never had a concept of ownership. Even once I arrived in England, I only had a handful of soft toys and while I never wanted for anything, my parents valued quality over quantity.

My childhood home was cluttered with paperwork and my parents were constantly working, but we always had enough of what we needed. Growing up in a home where nothing was bought in excess must have had an impact on me. Just as I had few toys, I never had loads of clothes either, but what I did have were quality pieces that I was always willing to share with my girlfriends. As a teenager, I started to shop in Oasis, which was a really grown-up shop at the time. I had a mock-crocodile trench coat, in the palest pastel green, which I wore for years, along with my favourite brown pea coat, which I treasured until I lost it in a nightclub (I was *devastated*).

My mum taught me to buy good-quality items, so when I shop now, I'm always thinking about how long that item will last.

I've always been more than happy to share my possessions, but I have also experienced the benefits of other people sharing with *me*. As my parents worked a lot, I would spend time at a neighbour's house after school. They had an open-door policy and their home was truly beautiful. It was full of Laura Ashley furniture and was cosy and organised – the exact opposite of my own home. While the *things* in that house were lovely, what I valued most was that my neighbours would share their time and food with me – their space and their love. I ate dinner with them most nights and spent several holidays with them.

As an adult, the values that are important to me now include having the ability to share your *space*. It's far more powerful than sharing things. So many times I've seen the value that inviting someone into your house can bring. When you can give someone a cuddle, a seat at the table or a bed, it outweighs any financial or physical help.

Through my work, I've seen so many people who have closed their doors to friendship and family because they are embarrassed of what their homes have become. Many people buy material objects because they believe it will make them happy, only to find they are drowning in them later on. They can't stop accumulating things and then they can't share their life, because they don't want others to see the mess they're in.

Time and space are the two most valuable commodities, but it seems that so many people struggle to share them. However, it's those elements that are often the things we crave most from other people.

If you're getting ready to share your space, before we talk practically, look inwards. Sharing can be a huge issue for many people. Unless you've grown up sharing your space, get ready for a significant impact on the way you live. Children with siblings might be more familiar with sharing and are often more relaxed about having a busy house. But only-children can find it harder, because they're simply not used to having to share. Before we begin this chapter, dig deep and work out whether you are the sort of person who is comfortable with sharing your things, your space and your time.

Collect
memories,
not
things.

KEY LIFE CHANGE

Think about it. All your friends want is to be able to come to your house, sit down and have a cup of tea with you. All your children want is to be able to play in a space that is free. All you want to do is get into your bed at the end of the day in a calm room. All of these things are just simple notions, aren't they?

Having your friends around for dinner, hosting your family at Christmas, having your grandchildren to stay or letting your kids have a sleepover. They are such normal, straight-forward activities... and they create an opportunity to make memories. If your house has been taken over by things, you can't spend time with your family or share your space.

When we look at sharing space, it's important to decide WHO we want to share that space with and WHY.

Use this motivation whenever you are flagging or feeling overwhelmed by the decluttering process.

Even when our neighbours pop round for a cup of tea or our kids have a playdate, we are sharing our space. That concept goes all the way through to moving in with a partner, having a baby, or a parent coming to live with you. But does sharing come naturally to you? If your child has a playdate, are you quick to invite the kids back to yours? Would you offer the plumber a cup of tea while they are sorting out your pipes?

The way you treat visitors is a reflection of your own ability to share.

MOVING IN WITH A PARTNER

If your first experience of sharing space will be moving in with a partner, ask yourself how you will *be* in that shared space? How will you *live* together?

In the bedroom, you'll need a chest of drawers, a wardrobe and possibly a bedside table each, but whatever furniture you bring in needs to be communal. If you don't do this, you'll set yourself up for arguments, so I suggest you start with a mindset of compromise.

Combine and reduce your belongings to fit the space you have so that it works for both of you.

In the kitchen, you don't need two of everything. Work out who has the best kettle, the best pans, the nicest cutlery. Keep only the best-quality pieces, or the ones in better condition. Sometimes starting afresh with nothing can be a way to save arguments as to who has the best

stuff, but remember that you never want to waste items that are of good quality and can still be used. Merging two households should always be led by prioritising quality along with considering the space you have available. Then donate or sell anything that you no longer need.

WELCOMING A CHILD

If you're welcoming a child into your home, be it a new baby or an older child, it's likely you're going to lose a spare bedroom. Perhaps you're sacrificing your walk-in wardrobe and feel panicked about the change. But if you've *chosen* to welcome a new addition to your family, it hopefully shouldn't feel like too much of a loss. A longed-for baby is a great reason to give up your excess shoes, clothes and handbags!

In any situation where you are changing your space, remind yourself why you're doing it.

Focus on the practicalities of working out how you are going to make the new space work. What furniture will you move? What storage can you invest in? Is it time to change your bed for one with built-in storage? Investigate containers to store out-of-season clothes and think about rotating your wardrobe seasonally. Maybe you can still keep a wardrobe in your baby's room, as a baby won't need much hanging space for the first year!

Alternatively, if your spare bedroom is currently your office, can you move your desk to the front room or find enough space on the landing? In shared living spaces, ask yourself if it's time to pack away your books or vinyl collection to make space for baby toys.

Whatever you decide to change, I'd like you to remember that it is only temporary. Just because you have someone new in your house, you don't have to lose your identity. Even if you do bring baby toys into a formerly adult space, you can retain your existing furniture.

When the child is old enough and doesn't need bulky toys any more, your vinyl can return to the sideboard. Any changes that allow you to share your space don't need to last forever.

Keeping baggage from the past will leave no room for happiness in the future.

Focus forwards

Keeping baggage from the past will leave no room for happiness in the future. If you are feeling overwhelmed because of the clutter, focus on what you want to achieve to keep you on track with getting your home ready to share. Remember your goals and think deeply about how you can create a shared space that will benefit you and those you love.

HOSTING VISITORS

Are you really ready to share? Embarrassment and shame can be huge barriers to letting other people into your life. If you want to open your house to others, you need to ask yourself some tough questions.

Some people are happy continuing to buy so much stuff that visitors can't get in, because deep down they don't *want* visitors. But I also work with many families who say, 'I'd love to share my house if only I had the space'. They *do* have plenty of space, but they can't open their doors because they have filled their home with clutter and they are too embarrassed to let visitors see.

A lot of people aren't natural givers and if you're truly happy like that, that's fine. Only you will know the kind of person you are, or who you want to become.

I know from personal experience that mental illness and distress can play a big part in individuals wanting to close their doors to others, but my career has also taught me that many people simply don't open their doors because of the state of their houses, not their hearts. They feel they can't have people round. When they understand the effects of decluttering, it's truly life-changing.

It's incredible to see that individuals who were formerly lonely now get regular visits from grandchildren, their oldest friends can now stay over, and they welcome family to a roast dinner around the dining table every Sunday. They now enjoy positive life-sharing experiences, whereas before they had a very insular existence.

'Maybe the life you've always wanted is buried underneath everything you own.'

Joshua Becker

THE BIG PICTURE

NOTHING'S FOREVER

As you move through life, sharing your space, you need to remember that nothing is permanent. So many people panic about change, but when you declutter and tidy, often all you are doing is returning your home to how you wanted it to be. Get back to the feeling that you have a beautiful house that people *want* to spend time in – a space that will make you feel calm and happy.

Once you have reintroduced structure to your home, all the turmoil that had been created will vanish.

If you ever feel as though you can't see the wood for the trees or get on top of everything, your mind will be edging towards chaos. Don't panic – this is *very* normal. Yes, you will have to work at setting some boundaries and getting things done, but then you will be able to appreciate your home again. And once you've broken your bad habits, your mental health will improve.

CHANGING YOUR ATTITUDE TO OWNERSHIP

It is also hugely beneficial to try to change your attitude to the concept of ownership. Do you really need to OWN everything that you need? I see it all the time, in people's need to buy a brand-new dress or suit for every special occasion, even though they know they will only wear it once. It's ridiculous! There are other options, especially if you know that you're not going to get much

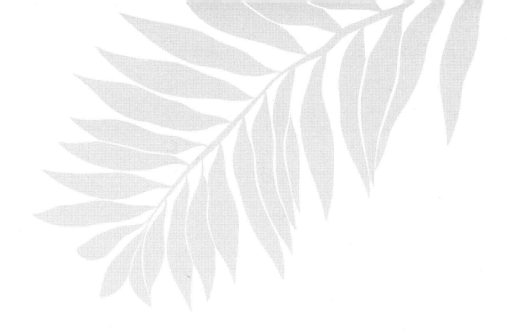

use out of something. People are gradually starting to come around to the idea of rental schemes. There are so many out there: clothing hire, toy libraries, tool libraries. Why buy an expensive sander or a carpet cleaner if you can rent one for a couple of days and then return it for the next person to use? This also extends to understanding that not everything in your own space has to be permanent.

Maybe I do what I do because I've never believed in ownership. I feel as though everyone is on borrowed time and every*thing* is borrowed. Nothing in our lives is long-term, so why do you feel you need ownership over items? Letting go of the notion that you have to own something and keep everything forever will make you feel so much better.

You don't *have* to own a house, or a toy, or a car. I know that people will find this concept hard, but you don't need to have possessions to validate yourself. Just because you haven't *bought* the dress, it doesn't mean that you don't look amazing in it. Just because you don't *own* your car, it doesn't mean you can't afford it. It just means you want to give it back at a later date. You will ultimately have a freer mindset if you embrace the concept of sharing.

It's better for the planet – and your home – if it's rented.

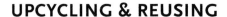

UPCYCLING & REUSING

As you consider switching up your space to share it with others, look at your furniture to see what you could repurpose in a different way or in a different room. I'm sure you have a piece of furniture lying around that could actually be used by someone else. Alternatively, if you need something new, does it have to be NEW – could you buy second-hand? Look at traditional items in a different way:

> Could you convert a vintage piece of furniture into toy storage? You don't have to use dedicated (and ugly) children's storage units – put toys in something nice to look at.

> If a drawer unit is falling apart, could you repurpose the drawers and use them as under-bed storage?

> Can you put up bookshelves to house your shoes?

> Do you have any old gift boxes that you're saving? They would be perfect storage for small items, such as make-up or tiny toys.

> Use your suitcases to store blankets and bedding while you're not on holiday to get maximum use from them – and have a tidier room.

> Outgrown children's wardrobes or old dressers can go into the garage to be used as storage for sport's equipment or tools.

> Old fitted kitchen cabinets and units are also great as repurposed storage in your utility room or garage.

> Old shoeboxes or Tupperware without lids can be used inside drawers as dividers and storage for smaller things.

LOOK AFTER YOURSELF

Learning to share is a key life skill. In Sri Lankan culture, it's considered rude if people come to your house and leave without eating. When I was a teenager, even though my parents were working, my mum would always cook for my friends. I'm the same now. It's common courtesy to offer a simple refreshment such as tea or coffee to guests, but I've worked in many houses where I haven't even been offered a glass of water. Conversely, in other homes, the owners have made sure I sit down at lunchtime and get a proper meal served on bone china! How you treat people in your home is such a show of character.

It also proves that sharing, even as an adult, is learned behaviour. If you see an action repeated, you will follow those patterns. Humans can't help but pick up bad habits

and when you're absorbing those methods, they'll come back to you as an adult. If you see your parents smoke, it's likely you are going to smoke too. If your parents are positive people, genuinely upbeat, you're likely to provide a similarly positive experience in your home. I believe it's so important to always lead by example.

When we were buying our house, in terms of aesthetics it wasn't our first choice, nor was it in my dream location, but it did have enough garden space for us to build in and it was walking distance to a high street. We had to sacrifice what we wanted as newlyweds for my mum's benefit.

My mum sacrificed her whole life for me. She travelled half-way round the world to find me! I might not be wild about my house, but I will always be

Childhood homes

**Think back and consider how you were brought up.
Your childhood experiences often have an effect on how you
keep your home today.**

Take your notebook and look at your home, then compare it to your parents' home. Write down all the similarities and differences you can think of in the two spaces. Are they the same or are they very different?

Next, list down what you learned from your parents. Make two columns for a list of things that you repeated from your childhood and a list of things you have actively tried to change or avoid.

You might want to think about whether your parents often had people round. How did those occasions feel? Now flip those questions around: what lessons are you teaching your children? What will your children say when they think back to their own childhoods?

Whether you have children or not, how would you like guests in your home to perceive you? How would you like them to feel – and how do you think they *actually* feel? Relaxed, comfortable and looked after, or nervous and on edge?

What would you like visitors to take away from their experience in your house?

able to sleep at night, knowing I did my best for my mum while she was here.

If you've come to the conclusion that you aren't sharing your space, but you'd like to or you need to, think about how you can improve things. This depends on how much effort you are willing to go to. What are you willing to sacrifice?

Maybe you want to clear that space to make it work for your parents to live with you, to welcome a baby or child into your family, or to entertain and give back to friends who've supported you.

Weigh up the compromises and take some time to analyse your motives before you begin to prepare the physical space.

Remember, you are in control of your space. You are in control of what you bring into your house.

'Out of clutter, find simplicity. From discord, find harmony. In the middle of difficulty lies opportunity.'

Einstein

WELLBEING BENEFITS

Humans need some sort of control in their lives. We may
not always be able to control our emotions or mental states, but our
homes are sometimes the only space we feel we *can* control. When
we walk out of our front doors, we can lose that control – anything
can happen – but our homes are our safe place. You can choose to
control what comes into your house; even taking back that small
amount of control will leave you starting to feel more positive.

So many people contact me and say that they know what they need
to do, they know what they want to achieve, but they just can't get
started without my professional help. Because they're drowning
in stuff, they can't remember the positive feeling that comes from
being tidy. They can't remember the feeling they had when they first
walked into their house and the space was clear. That feeling of calm
and clarity has been lost among clutter and chaos.

So, take a moment to consider your happy place. Think about the
feeling that you would like from your home. Tell yourself exactly how
you want to feel. If you are able to visualise it, you will get the feeling
back, I promise. Even if you know that the process is going to be
tough, having a clear-out will make you feel so much better.

How much do you want that change? If you want it, you will make it
happen.

You know that your house is going to look better and you will feel
better, but you need to transfer that feeling from your future into
the NOW.

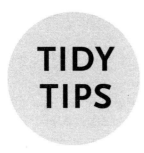

TIDY TIPS

LEAD BY EXAMPLE

If you're living in a shared space, focus on *your* space first. In a student house or flat-share, make sure your own space is as organised as it can be before you get involved with anyone else's space and possessions. Housemates will see how you are living and, hopefully, want to get involved in your calm, uncluttered existence. (Although sometimes they won't and you'll just have to let them be!) If you decide to reorganise the kitchen or tidy the living space, you need to check with other people first that it's okay. It's hard to live with other people's chaos if you're an organised person, but try to ignore others' clutter. I understand that can be really stressful, but be patient, until the people you live with are ready to get involved.

Families that I work with often complain that others in the family unit are the messy ones. They want to know how they can change them. But, by continuing to lead by example, you will be making changes that others can see the benefits of. Hopefully, before long they will be ready for you to show them the way.

Alternatively, you can take control and tidy for them (always ask first), but you might have to be prepared for the fact that they may not maintain your good work. But the hope is that they will see what you've done and the benefits of how it makes you feel.

They will see the positive change waiting for them and want to do it themselves.

A certain amount of selflessness is needed. I know a lot of people will ask, 'Why should I tidy up their mess?' Particularly parents, who end up tidying every single day and constantly picking up after everyone. One solution is implementing a really simple, accessible system for storage. With your kids' toys, make it really obvious where the Lego, the Playmobil, the dolls and the art equipment all go. Once you add labels, it's even easier. And the more they put things away themselves, the easier it is for that action to stick in their consciousness.

Structure will help you guide your family to be tidy and encourage them to put things back in the right place. Continue to lead by example. We can't expect our children's rooms to be tidy if our rooms aren't. If your kids can see you putting your clothes in the laundry basket, that will reinforce their behaviours as well. And remember: you can't expect your children to put their dirty clothes in a laundry basket if it's not easy to access. I gave Nelly a little basket of her own and, instead of chucking her school uniform on the floor, it now goes in the basket at the end of the day.

STRUCTURE

I think schools do an amazing job of teaching organisation because kids are not allowed to just chuck the toys back in any old drawer. There is a space for paper, a space for crayons... Everything's labelled to perfection and there is a rigid system. That's the sort of structure you need to bring into your home. Give your kids a place for their pencils. Make sure they have what they need, but no more. When we give our kids too much freedom and too much choice, we lose control.

When you're sharing a space with others, structure allows people to have their own personal space and identity.

People like ownership and, as I saw with my mum, they need their own private space. I go down to my mum's annexe every week to keep an eye on things. I always ask if she wants help tidying, because although it's her space to do what she wants with, she has poor mental health so she does need constant care.

Because we reduced the amount she has to deal with on a daily basis – she's no longer surrounded by unnecessary things – it's easier for her to maintain, which makes the space feel like hers to own. But I still need to keep on top of things. More often than not, I will just pop in and work on whatever areas I think need attention, despite my mum's comments on what I'm doing and why I'm doing it!

FOCUS ON ONE TASK AT A TIME

Whenever you take on a tidying job, it's important to take it task by task. Multitasking, working on different rooms and areas at the same time, will *not* help you to focus. Think clearly and focus on one area.

Choose a smaller space first and it will feel less overwhelming.

Saying to yourself, 'I'm going to sort the garage/playroom/kitchen today' can sometimes be too much of an expectation – you might not finish the task and then feel disheartened. But if you break things down into smaller elements, even if you only recycle six Nurofen syringes today, that's an achievement.

Small tasks are both manageable and achievable. When you have a win – however small – it's still a win. And that gives you a mental boost and a sense of accomplishment. Even cleaning the cutlery drawer will give you a sense of achievement, as would clearing out your make-up bag. Tomorrow morning, when you put your make-up on, that freshened bag will make the process feel lovely.

Try to build up your small wins every day. Start with a 15-minute task, then try two. Before you know it, you could find yourself on a three-hour tidying session! The sense of achievement grows and grows until your whole house is immaculate.

10 QUICK WINS

Choose one 15-minute task to focus on each day to stop
you feeling overwhelmed. Break areas down into sections – they're
much easier to tackle this way.

1. Match up all the Tupperware lids and containers in the kitchen
   cupboard.

2. Do the same with your pots and pans: make sure you know
   which lid matches which pan.

3. Gather up all the toys and playthings that aren't where they
   should be and put them back in their relevant tubs and boxes
   (Lego in the Lego box, and so on...).

4. Clean out the cutlery drawer and put everything back in
   designated sections.

5. Recycle all the medicine syringes in the cutlery drawer.

6. Clear out your make-up bag and wash all your make-up brushes.

7. Go through the medicine cabinet and take all out-of-date
   products to a pharmacy to dispose of safely.

8. Clear out the old receipts from your purse/wallet. Recycle those
   you no longer need and file the ones you must keep.

9. Go through memory boxes and get rid of anything that no
   longer triggers emotion.

10. Look at your underwear drawer and recycle anything past its
    best, anything stained or with holes, or single socks.

SEASONAL PLANNER
Summer

Summer is the best time to look at your outdoor space. These are the months – weather permitting – when it's easier to forget about your inside space because you will be living outside more. The windows are open, the doors are open and we're all looking outwards, rather than inwards.

Sunny weather gives you the best opportunity to make big changes in your garden, or to organise large outdoor storage areas, such as sheds or garages.

If your goal is to share your space socially, you might be planning on making an entertaining zone outside – perhaps building a bar or a lovely barbecue or seating area that family and friends can enjoy.

It's very easy to forget about your outside area as a way to create more space within your house. External socialising spaces mean you're not messing up your inside rooms.

Consider investing in external storage to house items you don't need in the house all year round.

If you don't have a garden, garage or shed, don't just see this as an opportunity to take a rest from the decluttering – choose another area instead (I suggest the utility room, see page 92) and get ahead!

BIG SPACE 1: GARAGE/SHED

I find that the problem with garages and sheds is that they often just turn into a dumping ground – the place where we shove everything that doesn't have a proper home. Most of the time you don't know where anything is because you're just trying to climb through all the stuff! And when you need to find something specific, like a screwdriver, you've got no idea where it is because there's sports equipment, lawnmowers and toys that never made it to the charity shop clogging up the space. I often feel that our garages and sheds

DOLLY DASH 1

Paint store

Summer is a great time to Dolly Dash your paint store. I know you have one! Give yourself 15 minutes to gather up all the old paints in your shed, then take them to a dump or recycling centre where they can be safely disposed of. Some recycling centres even offer paint reuse facilities, where people can pick up half-used cans for free, to complete small decorating projects.

Go through your paint brushes and rollers and if there are any brushes with bristles coming out, find a way to recycle them. Make sure any items that you decide to keep are clean, dry and in good enough condition to use again.

Next, use containers, whether that's new plastic crates or old shoe boxes, to split up the paint-brushes and rollers (as well as keeping separate boxes for other tools, such as wallpaper scrapers or screwdrivers). Separating your belongings into as many containers as you can will help anyone into DIY stay organised.

(and lofts and spare rooms) are full of decisions we simply can't bring ourselves to make.

Clutter is nothing more than postponed decisions.

Garages and sheds are so often used as overflow and, although I realise that this space can be essential if you have a large family as it lets you save money on storage, I'd like to remind you that you shouldn't feel that you automatically have to fill this space up. I'm also not keen on encouraging overflow – you should try to contain all of your belongings in their own dedicated space. But if you really, *really* need some extra room, then these places are very useful to store items you only need seasonal access to.

Before you start to bring anything out of your shed or garage, the most important thing is to decide whether you have got the right structure in place for putting everything back in an organised manner. Perhaps you need racking or shelves. Do you need some large stackable containers? You might have several bikes, so do they need bike racks?

Ensure you have the correct storage purchased and ready in advance so that you can organise all the items you keep in these spaces back into dedicated sections.

Choose a dry, warm day to get everything out of your shed or garage to assess it. I always encourage you to empty all of your belongings out and go through absolutely everything. Choose dry weather as you want to ensure nothing gets damaged or starts to go rusty during the process. Lay everything out on the ground and divide it all into groups. This will allow you to assess exactly what you still need to keep – and what you don't.

Useful groupings:

> Gardening tools

> DIY tools

> Outdoor activities (games equipment)

> Beach equipment

> Hobby equipment (bikes, scooters)

> Outdoor entertaining accessories (barbecue/barbecue accessories/umbrella/gazebo/deckchairs/loungers/outdoor occasional chairs/seasonal lights)

> Paint

> Outdoor cleaning equipment

> Camping equipment

The best way to put each of these groupings back in an organised way is to plan your storage first.

What would be the best way to arrange all these items? Is it in boxes or crates, or on racking? What size storage do you need? Consider small tubs for screws and nails, and larger boxes for camping equipment. Make sure everything you're putting back works and is in good condition, ready for when you want to use it again. Anything that you no longer need could be donated to a tool library or charity shop.

BIG SPACE 2: UTILITY ROOM

You don't need to wait for a sunny, dry day to get involved with clearing out your utility room, but if you do have access to an outside area, it helps to physically spread out your items. Take everything out of the room, clear every cupboard and drawer, and then give the space a thorough clean.

Go through all the items that were in the room and group them. Everything needs to be kept with similar items so it will be easy to find what you're looking for. Ideas for groupings include:

> Laundry equipment (iron and pegs)

> Laundry supplies (detergent bottles and packets)

> Cleaning appliances and equipment (dusters, cloths, brushes, hoover and mop)

> Cleaning products (bottles and packets)

> Shoe-cleaning supplies

> Batteries

TOY ROTATION

If you have too many kids' toys in the house, you could consider using the garage or shed as a place to store and rotate them. This has the benefit of keeping your living spaces clearer, and your kids aren't swamped by the amount they have. Toys can be stored in the garage quite happily and get swapped over when the kids are bored with their current selection.

Kids often get sensory overload and feel overwhelmed by too many toys; it's easy to assume that they need lots, but actually they don't. Kids go through so many phases – what they play with changes constantly. If you can store the toys and bring something old back into circulation as 'new', it will stop you needing to buy something brand new (or finding a place to get rid of something old). It makes so much sense to pack away some toys and start rotating them during the summer months, as you'll find your kids are playing outside more.

If, during this process, you find toys that have been outgrown or are definitely not played with any more, donate or sell those that are still in good condition and throw away those that are not. Don't keep them!

A word of warning: if you're packing toys away and tidying, try to do it at a time when your children are at a playdate or at school. If you start to pack away toys while they are around, your kids might suddenly rediscover their old favourites and want to bring them *all* back into the house – then you're back to square one!

> Lightbulbs

> Paper towels

> Vases

As you're going through the items, ask whether there are any items in your utility room that don't belong there. Where *should* they live? Go and put them back in the right place, so they don't clog up the dedicated utility space.

With each group of items, look at what you have. Do you have duplicates? Are there similar items? Your goal is to reduce what you need, so if you find you have three glass vases that are all the same, donate two to the charity shop.

When it's time to return all the items back into the space, before you bring them in, you need to contain them. By containing items you will make sure that you don't overbuy again (because you have a visual of the space that item can fill) and you will also stay organised when it comes to using those things in the future. Labelling the containers is also very helpful. Now, neatly slot in the containers and your utility room will be done.

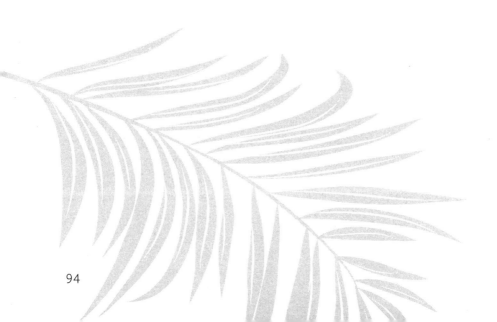

DOLLY DASH 2

Cleaning supplies

I often see people who live in small spaces bulk-buying cleaning products. They don't have space for them and they won't ever use them! Cleaning products are a great area to Dolly Dash. See if you can reduce your stash to only keep the products you use every day and fit them into just one container or caddy.

I only use five cleaning products: limescale remover, polish, anti-bac spray, some bleach and a multi-purpose spray for kitchen and bathroom surfaces. These all fit into one caddy and any dusters, cloths or brushes can be slotted into a Tupperware box and kept next to the products.

I advise keeping containers under your sink for your specialist products (such as dishwasher tablets or washing powder), and keeping the caddy under there too.

If you have more time, consider your laundry. If you don't have an outside area to dry your clothes, could you find some wall space to put up a retractable washing rack or can you put up a couple of hooks to store a clothes horse? This could save you having to drape laundry on radiators around the house, creating a calmer living space on laundry days.

LIFE LESSON

The most common problem that I come across with sharing space is when children have to share a room. I've seen so many children that never get to express their own identity within a room.

One family I worked with had two boys and two teenage girls, and those four children shared two rooms. The girls got on with each other, which helped, but they still needed to have their own space. In this case, the solution was to create a room within a room. We started by thinking of the room as two halves, rather than a whole, and configured it to create an individual, cosy room for one of the girls within the space. You could use bookshelves to divide a room, but if you're handy, you can make very inexpensive MDF walls to create this extra area, which is what we did. She now has a cabin-style bed with walls around it and a curtain that can be closed when she's watching TV (I hung the TV on the wall to make extra space). By looking at the space as two rooms, I could see a way to equally divide it, so both girls could have the same amount of furniture (such as beds, wardrobes, chests of drawers and bedside tables).

The boys' room remained as a whole but we made each section of the room reflect their individual personalities. When each child looked around their side of the room, they could immediately see they were surrounded by things that reflected their likes and hobbies – and not what their brother was into! It's a really important visual effect to try to create in a shared space, to make sure each child has their own personality expressed. Whether you are dividing a room for boys or girls, paint the walls different colours to give each person their own identity within the space.

Another family that I worked with had two boys who had separate rooms, but in a configuration that still wasn't working. One boy was in a box room with literally just a bed, while the other was in a large room, surrounded by toys. They also wanted to sleep in the same room, so it made more sense to let them share the bigger room and create a toy room. The result was that both boys now have equal amounts of living space, equal amounts of furniture (including a desk) and they can play together happily, too. They have a better quality of living space from the changes we made.

In both cases, looking at the floorplan of the houses – and avoiding the constraints of allocating a space as a bedroom, just because it's upstairs – was key.

Sharing your space means constantly asking what sort of quality of life and living space the people in your house have. Are they comfortable in that space? Can they be moved to another room, a bigger room? Would swapping rooms create a better space and a better way of living?

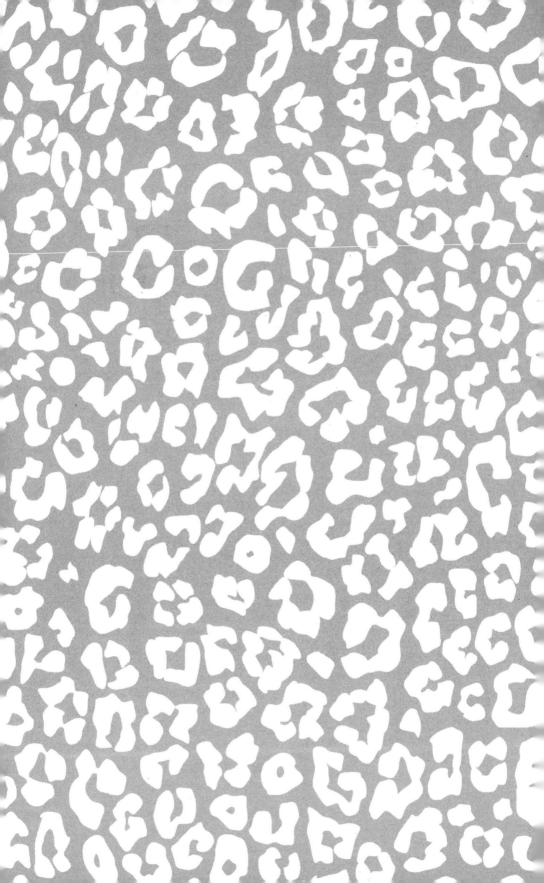

PART THREE

CHANGE
your view

CHANGE (verb), 1: make someone or something different; alter or modify; **2:** replace something with something else, especially something of the same kind that is newer or better; substitute one thing for another.

MY STORY

My mum and dad were well into their forties and fifties when they adopted me. I was a three-year-old girl from another country, who had lived in an orphanage all her life and been brought up by nuns. I only spoke Sri Lankan and I had never eaten English food.

While it was obviously a big change for me, the change for them was immense too. So often we think only about the birth of a newborn baby as something that triggers change in our homes, but my whole life changed when I was adopted. Similarly, my parents had to adapt everything they'd done for half their lives on the day I arrived. Sometimes, we go through our lives and are content with our routine, but life-changing events – planned or unplanned – mean we *have* to change.

I'd like you to remember that change isn't just about space either. Change affects how we evolve as people, too. It can alter us in so many ways and that has a knock-on effect on how we live in our homes, as well as what we think we need.

More and more families, like my parents, are adopting children at all ages from toddlers to teenagers. Those that foster have to adapt to huge ongoing changes too. As well as basic things like making sure there are enough beds in the house and making sure the home works for everyone in the household, foster parents need to try to create a welcoming home environment. That can be really hard to deal with, because everyone's life is turned upside down, even if it is only just for a short period of time.

However, as I said in the last chapter, it's good to keep in mind that all these life stages are temporary.

I often reflect on how the huge changes I've lived through in my life have affected me.

Am I good at decluttering because I lived my first three years with nothing? I also grew up in a chaotic environment and I often see people who repeat the same chaos in their own houses, or become the polar opposite – like me. As an adopted child, I was always curious to know if there was another family out there that was similar to mine, where an older couple had adopted a child from overseas (like me), as well as wondering if I had any biological brothers and sisters and how they were living. It's something I still want to discover. I kept in touch with the nuns from the orphanage. When I was getting married and needed to get hold of my birth certificate, Sister Bernadette told me that she knew someone who could help me get it. I thought this would be the perfect opportunity to take Charley to Sri Lanka.

I always believed that I was adopted because I was born out of wedlock. The story went that my birth mother was 17 when she met an English guy and had a fling. I was given up for adoption and that was it, apparently, but I was always curious to know more. When I arrived on the island, the fixer told me he could also reconnect me with my birth mother. I had two days to decide whether I wanted to meet the person who changed the course of my life all those years ago! I had to say yes.

The woman I met only spoke Sri Lankan. She had a good job in the local government office and I learned that she had married and adopted her own child. However, 30 years on, my existence is still a secret to all beyond her closest family. It turned out that my father was known (so, *not* a fling). He died the same year as my adopted dad, 2010, which was rather a coincidence. Apparently, he took his own life as he had cancer and couldn't afford the treatment. The woman was crying, sobbing and saying sorry throughout our time together but, and it's the weirdest thing, when I left the meeting Charley and I both said, 'Imagine if it's *not* her'. I felt no connection with her whatsoever. After the meeting, she emailed me to tell me she had no money and asked if I could bring her to live in England. We've never spoken again and I never replied to that email. I still doubt that she was my real mother. How do I know it was really her? It could have been a scam. I'm not even sure if the name on the birth certificate is mine. Only a DNA test could tell the truth. I've learned first-hand that change can come at us from every angle, at any stage of our lives.

GRIEF AND CHANGE

In order for change to be effective, you *have* to make a considered choice. But there are times when you can't plan for change. Maybe you're getting divorced or a relative has died. Changing while you're dealing with grief is the hardest. We experienced this when Charley's mum died in a car crash. The family had two weeks to clear out his late-mum's home – they had no choice. It didn't matter that she had lived there for years, that she was a mother, a grandmother, an aunt, a friend. All that mattered was that the council needed the house for a new family, and that was that.

Sometimes, your only choice is to deal with a situation and do it fast (if there is a time limit, for example). Speed, however, can also have a detrimental effect – for example, if you've been forced to make decisions when you haven't had time to grieve. Charley and his family cleared the whole house, but none of them could face emptying the sink... It still had all the washing-up in it from the day that she died. Charley's mum had left the house to go to work, thinking she'd come back and do the dishes, but she never came home. For Charley and his family, that was the hardest part of the process.

Being creatures of habit is something that none of us acknowledge until we realise that something has to change because there is an element of our lives that is making us miserable. Work out what the problem is, ask yourself who the problem is affecting, then decide what you need to change and why that change is necessary. When a situation starts disturbing the relationships around you, that's a sign that you have to knuckle down and work to bring change into your life. Whether the catalyst is of your own making, or something outside of your control, you might go through a different process to deal with it, but the result – change – remains the same.

I've learned first-hand that change can come at us from every angle, at any stage of our lives.

Throughout the different stages of my life, many of which might echo changes you too will go through, I always think about how I can adapt the process of change to benefit me. If you do want to undertake change in your home, the goal is always to make the space flow better. But there's no point doing something quickly and hoping for the best. You need to plan.

Humans don't like change, but – once you get through it – it can be hugely beneficial.

Deep down, particularly when things aren't going our way, we know that something's gotta give. In terms of clutter, it's only when our kitchen becomes so chaotic that we can't function in it, that we realise something's *got* to change. When you continue living in a pattern, repeating what you've always done, you'll never come to realise the benefits of a new way of life.

KEY LIFE CHANGE

Welcoming someone into your home is always about self-sacrifice, whether it's a temporary guest or a new baby. As I discussed in the last chapter, it's really important to identify what you are *really* like as a person. Change often requires us to be selfless, so you need to ask yourself, what are you capable of sacrificing, in order to achieve what you want?

BLENDING FAMILIES

Maybe you're blending your families together – you've got three kids from one relationship and your partner has two kids from their previous relationship. If you can only afford a three-bedroom house and have five kids, it's basic maths that the children are going to have to share! Your decision to join your families together depends on how much

you want to be together, as well as how you're going to physically split up a house. If you're going for it, you will have to make sacrifices and compromises.

Once you know that the kids will be sharing, it's time to decide how you are going to make this situation work best. Cramming two families' belongings into one space is going to be tough, so you could look at your joint finances and see if you're able to move house. I encourage you to list your requirements to make sure you know what sort of house you might be looking for, whether that's something with more living space or another bedroom. Bear in mind that, even if you can't move, there are plenty of ways to make your current living space more pleasurable. I suggest that you start by looking for inspiration in magazines, online and on social media to find houses and rooms that are similar to yours that you like, and look for ways you can recreate that in your own home.

EMBRACING PERSONAL IDENTITIES

Sometimes you don't have a lot of choice. And that lack of choice can leave you feeling stuck. Taking away choice feels like taking away a person's identity. If you can't get more space, you will have to come up with some creative solutions instead. A lot of the houses I go into have rooms with absolutely no identity. It's important to work on giving personality to shared living spaces. I often see children's rooms with no identity, but it's vital to give kids an opportunity to showcase their personalities, likes and dislikes, even if they are sharing a space.

If you put several kids in one bedroom, I encourage you to think about how they can each have their own identity in that room. Is it possible? Sometimes it's not, but splitting the space equally is a great place to start. Give each child a side of the room to call their own and work with them, if they are old enough, to make sure that the areas are visually different. Let them choose different paint colours or wallpapers, or even different furniture and headboards, if you can. Allow them to pick something in the room that they can use to identify the space as *theirs* rather than a shared space. Encourage them to choose posters for the walls that reflect their individual interests and hobbies.

Consider how the room is working and if it's doing its job effectively. Does everyone sharing that space have the right sort of storage and is it shared out equally? If the kids have a communal wardrobe, ensure they have an equal amount of stuff in it.

IT'S GOOD TO TALK

I always want to motivate you to consider what you are willing to sacrifice for the wonderful change that lies ahead.

Think of the non-negotiables for your entire family and keep in mind that this may be a short-term situation. If you know you're moving into a period of adjustment that means undertaking change for no more than six months, consider how you can make your space a transitional place. I suggest you do that by looking forward to the moment when you can change your space again. But instead of just flipping it back to how it was, think about what you would do differently. You've had the chance to live in a different way, so think about how the space has functioned in this transitional period. Has it actually been brilliant, so good you're considering changing it permanently? Or do you now realise exactly what you're missing in your home and can work out what you need to do once the transitional period is through?

Sometimes it's hard, but I would like you to remember that any tricky conversations should take place early on in the process, so you – and your family – can plan around the change and decipher the best ways to adapt your home for everyone that will live there.

TAKE CONTROL

Sometimes there are choices you are able to take charge of. Perhaps you're making the decision to have a baby, adopt a child or bring someone to live in your house. But when it comes to the changes that you wouldn't have made or that have been forced upon you, think of ways in which you can regain the power in those choices. I think you can still feel positive about changes that you're not in control of by taking control of what you're going to do in your space. You should never feel that there is only one way. I want to encourage you to always remember that *you* are in control of your space, even if it's being impacted by a life change that you didn't want.

Remember that YOU are in control of your space and how you deal with it.

DEALING WITH BEREAVEMENT

You might be facing a loved one's death within your household, or dealing with the aftermath of someone dying and leaving you a house to clear. In both circumstances, there is no finite advice that anyone can give you when you are faced with bereavement. There are no clear-cut answers and there is no timeline. We know that grief has no end – it just changes shape – so it's essential that you make sure that you are doing things at your own pace.

There is never a right or wrong answer to the way that a grieving person deals with something. When you are faced with living in a place that is full of memories of that person, you have to do what feels right at that time. I implore you not to rush and not to let anyone else tell you what to do. Do whatever you need to, in your own time.

After my dad died, my mum could never bring herself to sleep in their bed again. She went to sleep in the spare room, on the bed where the cat always slept – it's what she had to do to cope with his passing. Even when Mum moved out of the house, she chose never to sleep in a double bed again. You will know that grief can affect people very differently and please remember that it's okay *not* to be okay.

Sometimes it's okay just to exist.

I often get calls requesting my help from women who tell me their husband died five years ago and they still don't know how to deal with his belongings. It takes time. If you have acknowledged that you need some change and had a realisation that you need to get some of the space in your home back, then you will do it. But take it slowly. Don't rush. Start by working out what is affecting your daily life.

How can you reduce the things that are affecting you, to improve your own life right now?

Steps to your goal

**Use your notebook to write down a numbered list from 1 to 10.
Write your decluttering goal in at number 10.**

Instead of thinking of the goal as the ultimate 'to do', fill in each of
the other numbers with the steps and actions that will get you to
your final goal. This way, you'll feel less overwhelmed and can see
the route ahead – breaking down each step into smaller actions that
won't overwhelm you, or whoever you're encouraging.

For example, if you need to clear a garage, action point 1 will be
planning your storage, whether that's building shelves or buying
racks, as well as organising enough containers. 2) Pick a sunny day.
3) Plan how you're going to dispose of what you're removing. Is
there a recycling point or dump nearby or can you order a Hippo bag
or skip? 4) Work out whether you need help to clear the space (do
you need to employ a handyman for the day or can you work alone?).
5) Physically empty the space. 6) Group all the tools into their
sections, including items you need to dispose of. 7) Clean out the
shed or garage. 8) Begin to put everything back into containers.
9) Put the containers back into the garage on the nice, neat shelving
you planned at step number 1. Finally, you've reached your goal at
number 10 of 'clearing the garage' through a very manageable process.

Seeing your goal written down will also give you focus and help to
motivate you through the preceding steps.

THE BIG PICTURE

I wish I could suggest solid solutions that guaranteed that if you do *this*, you will live happily ever after, but I can't. Everything's a process. You need to work through every stage of change methodically and stay committed to your cause. You also need to understand why others in your home might be resistant to change and work through those issues together.

Most people resist change because it seems like too much of a challenge and it feels way out of their comfort zone. Tread carefully. Nothing is worse than arguing with someone who can't see, or won't accept, that change is necessary. Try to find some common ground – one thing that you may be able to agree on – and slowly, start changing small areas day by day, piece by piece.

Many people need to see the end result – the goal – before they invest in change, so find ways to show examples to them. Collate images, retell stories and do whatever you can to convince them. Unfortunately, some people won't change, particularly if you are navigating around grief, but *you* can change. If you consistently do what you believe in, others will hopefully see how important the change is to your relationship and to the way that they live in the home. Implement change gently without making it a big deal, slowly chipping away at things and continuing to gently encourage the process.

A little progress every day adds up to big results.

Little and often

Always start small and set short time limits so that the decluttering process is more manageable. It's key that you don't get overwhelmed and go into freeze mode where you're too panicked to do anything. Use the principle of a Dolly Dash and aim to complete small tasks. Don't plan on spending a whole day clearing the entire house. Start with 15 minutes. Work up to an hour. Pace yourself to reach half a day.

If you're struggling to decide where to start, choose the area that needs it most. What do you feel most overwhelmed by? Also consider what is manageable in the time you have. Perhaps you will dedicate your 15 minutes to a pile of toys on the floor or the books that never made their way back to the shelf. Think about doing each element in small stages, so it feels more manageable. Group all the Lego together, then go through the figures. Or start with puzzles today, then tomorrow move on to board games.

If you're working around the change that comes from ending a relationship or being bereaved, the most important thing is that you do it at your own pace (unless you are facing an obvious time constraint, as Charley and his family did). You might think, 'I can't make *any* decisions right now,' but follow the method of a space audit (see page 20) and go through the entire property, starting at the front door and working through it room by room, and it will soon be clear which things stand out as must-keeps, as well as those you're not bothered about and can get rid of immediately.

Remember to also come up with a solution about where the items you're removing will go.

Have you got enough space at home to rehouse a whole lifetime of stuff? It's unlikely. Often, when parents die, their children end up taking all their old furniture into their own homes. And there it stays, piled up, because they don't feel ready to go through it. Don't begin unless you're truly ready, but when you are, remember that you are trying to filter down these countless things to a small selection of items that *really* matter *and* that you've got space for. It's also worth considering whether the stuff you're bringing into your home is going to affect your own relationships.

It might sound odd, but don't forget that you don't actually have to keep anything physical. You don't need to save anything if you have wonderful memories. It's the same with children when we are building memory boxes. You may save your kids' first lock of hair or baby band from the hospital, or perhaps kept their first outfit or first blanket. But you certainly don't need to keep 14 different babygros, or every single scribble they ever did on the back of an envelope.

I've found through my work and in my own life that multiples of things don't matter or hold the same significance when you go back through those memory boxes 10 years later. So, when you *do* save particularly special items, it's important that you return to them and reassess them at regular intervals.

You can't reach for anything new if your hands are still full of yesterday's belongings.

While these are essential, practical tips to undertake, you need to ensure that you're not dealing with death or divorce on your own. Have you got support? Are your friends and family with you? Maybe you need paid support from someone completely impartial so that while you're looking after the non-negotiable items, they will box up the rest. Maybe you will keep five or six things that are absolutely essential, but there will also be plenty of items that you absolutely can't decide on now, so they should go to a temporary home while the rest of the items can go for good.

If you can visualise the positives that the things you're discarding can bring, it will make it so much easier. Think about the benefits of the discarded items to others if you are donating them or selling them. Think about the benefit to your inner calm if you no longer have to deal with too much furniture or sentimental items.

MAKE A FUTURE PLAN

I tell Charley all the time that if something happens to me, I want him to keep my jewellery for Nelly-Reet and everything else can go. It might sound morbid, but having open communication about these things will ease the practical aftermath of a death.

Make sure that your loved ones know what you want them to keep — and what you're not bothered about.

My mum is now 82 and she's looking more and more frail, although she could live another 20 years. Every time I see her walk up the garden path, I'm reminded that this could be her last year. You just don't know what is going to happen in the future, do you? So speak to your family about what will benefit you all now, while you can enjoy life together. Then think about who you want to be, moving forward. Ask why the things you have in your house are necessary and if they are helping you all, as a family, to enjoy your precious time together.

LOOK AFTER YOURSELF

THINKING AHEAD ABOUT DEATH

When a person passes away, I've got to warn you, there will be a point where emotion overtakes your thinking, however practically you've planned ahead. That's really tough. Everything that you *think* you want to do around their death might not happen as you planned because grief makes you lose sense of what needs to be done. But if you have general plans in place now, if you've already had open conversations about belongings, it *will* help in the long run.

As well as applying this thinking to close relatives, apply it to yourself. Think about what you are attaching your sense of self to, so that in the event of your death or serious illness your family doesn't have to

make difficult decisions or second-guess what you'd want when they're in the midst of grief or worry. If you've told them your wishes and they have taken them on board, at least you're not putting the burden of decision-making on them. You know the conversations I mean – whether you want to go into a home or can't bear the idea of sheltered accommodation, for example. It's definitely something that none of us want to talk about, but it will affect us all.

You don't have to ask others brutal questions, but you can ask them to share what are the most important things to them. Ask their thoughts on organ donation and how they would like to be remembered. Find out whether your relatives have a will or a plan. If you know something is really important to them, ask which family member they would like it to be passed on to. This is especially important if there are siblings involved.

As humans, as family members, we often struggle with the guilt attached to difficult decisions, but I believe that the problems – and the attached guilt – stem from the fact that we don't know the 'right' answer. If you have sat down with your parents, or other family members, and asked them their wishes outright, you will be free of that guilt in future (if you choose to honour their plans, of course!).

That's why it's important to have those conversations early on so that your parents can tell you that their books mean nothing and they're happy to send them to the library. Or they'll share that their furniture was really cheap so they'd rather you got rid of it all (before pointing out that there is one painting they think should be kept in the family). When we think about the physical things that connect us to a person, more often than not there will only be a handful of items. Think about your own parents and their house right now. What items remind you of your mum or your dad? It probably isn't a stack of books. My dad died

in 2010 and all that my mum chose to remind her of him was a very thin blue cushion, which my dad always used to sit on. That's just one item.

If you think about it, so many links to our loved ones are better stored in our memories, aren't they?

Communication is key. As well as talking with your family about the future, it's crucial that you also communicate truthfully with yourself. Keep checking in and reminding yourself to ask questions about what you're doing with the things you own, how you're approaching your home now and how that will change in the future.

Ultimately, by reminding yourself about who you are as a person, and deciphering what you want from your life, it will help you get the most out of every moment, as well as unravelling what it is that you want to be remembered for.

DEALING WITH UNWANTED CHANGE

Have you ever been made redundant? It's awful. And why is it so awful? Because no one gave you a choice. Maybe you would have chosen voluntary redundancy, but you weren't given an option. None of us get married with the future goal of getting divorced, do we? We get married because we want to stay married. So, if divorce hits you without it being your decision, the feelings you'll be going through revolve around the fact that you didn't want this change. You didn't *choose* to change. When you find out your partner has had an affair and they've left you, that already horrible situation is amplified because you didn't want that change. Someone else made a decision in which you had no say, yet it changes your whole life.

If you've been thrown into that situation and find yourself in the horrible place where you need to look at another house, change your car or how you live, you're having to take yourself out of your comfort zone. You'll be making decisions that you never wanted to even begin to contemplate, let alone go through with. Whether the situation is down to your own issues or completely not your fault, your discomfort boils down to the fact that you never wanted change. This may be coupled with the fact that you now have to make decisions jointly with someone that you don't see eye to eye with. It's never easy. Even if you're the happiest you could be, or you're having the most amicable divorce ever, or even if the divorce was your choice, there's always going to be *something*.

It's essential that you're ready for all the upcoming decisions and can prioritise what you need to get from the circumstances. Ask yourself, 'How can I make the very best of an awful situation?' I always felt that in the face of divorce, it is beneficial to start afresh – go back to the beginning and only think about what you absolutely need to take with you to *exist*. Obviously, there are huge financial considerations and I completely understand that some people have to take what they can, but I've always been fiercely independent, so I like to think that I could walk out of our house with my daughter (and the dog) and begin again. I also believe that my opinion stems from my mindset of never needing *things* or *stuff* around me, so I'm not emotionally attached to anything in my house. A big part of the problem, if you're going through a separation or dealing with death, is that you become attached to things because you bought them and used them *together*. But with any difficult situation, remember that *you* can make the decisions. *You* are in charge.

While you might not have chosen the situation, you can choose how it ends.

It's only when you've realised that change has to happen that you will be ready to take action.

Along with owning the responsibility that everything in your house is ultimately down to you, you have to own your responsibility for change, too. However hard other people might try, no one can force you to make any changes unless you are absolutely ready. If you're changing things before you've accepted the

WELLBEING BENEFITS

I promise you: so many wonderful things can happen once you are ready to accept change and go with it. Change will allow you to see your life from a new point of view. You can confront your demons and move on from them. Alternatively, change can let you step out of your comfort zone and achieve things you never thought you could. By spending time in self enquiry, constantly questioning how you're going to deal with change and getting ready to embrace it, change can improve your life and wellbeing in so many brilliant ways.

You know, some people will follow me for years, they'll listen to my Sunday sermons every single week, they'll like all my posts, but they are still not ready to make their own decisions about change. However, I have faith that one Monday they will wake up and think, 'Today's the day. I'm ready. I'm going to go for it.'

reasons *why* you have to change, that is when it can get uncomfortable. This is simply because you're not going at your own pace. That's when things won't feel as smooth as they should and you will start to resent the process.

Don't be deterred by the unsteady path of change. Don't ever let the uncertainty of the outcome stop you from trying, because it's only outside your comfort zone that great things happen. Focus on what you know you can achieve. I also recommend you get a positivity pad or set of affirmation cards to help you – something that will encourage you on every day of your journey.

PUT YOUR STAMP ON IT

If you've been forced into making a change that you didn't want, I'm going to give you one way you can make it feel more positive. Think about how you can bring your own personal signature to a space, whether it's reworking somewhere new or starting out on your own.

I would encourage you to remember what you love and work out what your personal style is. I always start by thinking about who my celebrity crush would be. Who would you most like to emulate, in terms of their style and interior aesthetic? I'm more Thandiwe Newton than Nicole Scherzinger, for example. I also love leopard print and have what I'd describe as a funky style. In brand terms, the look of my house is much more Rockett St George than Laura Ashley, because it's eclectic yet glam. A bit mix and match. So, if *you* are starting again, think about what you truly love so you can create a home that is a reflection of what you enjoy being surrounded by. If you are fresh out of a relationship, you may have made some decisions swayed by what the other person liked in order to please them (as we do in so many relationships). But now, enjoy the fact that you can choose your own style and you are completely in charge of your own decisions.

When starting again, think about what you truly love and create a home that is a reflection of what you enjoy being surrounded by.

Collate your taste

This is an exercise for your notebook or perhaps a Pinterest board.

Start by saving images of rooms, pictures of furniture or even colour combinations that you like and consider why you like them.

Get into the habit of justifying the reasons why they resonate with you and then work out how you can apply those inspiring ideas to your own home.

Consider how you can make changes that reflect the spaces you like. Where can you bring in these ideas?

How can you translate something that you admire in someone else's home into something more your style?

Clearing a loved one's house

Some people really struggle with making decisions in this situation, so begin with clearing the items that *are* easy to make a decision over. Create two piles and remember that you are getting ready to look at everything again later so nothing's set in stone:

Pile 1: Non-negotiables = items you feel sentimental about, the things you love the most, the things you simply have to keep.

Pile 2: Negotiables = everything else.

You'll find that quite soon you are filtering out things that you've realised you don't need. Everyone is different, so your non-negotiable item might be a beaten-up saucepan that your mum cooked the gravy for Sunday lunch in. She might have loved the process of welcoming her family into her home, and that pan – and the gravy – signified so many happy family memories. In which case, you save the pan and can make a final decision at a later date, when you're ready. Conversely, your mum might have hated that pan because the gravy always stuck to the bottom, in which case it's easy to get rid of.

Don't think of your piles as being a definite 'keep' or 'throw', or a straightforward 'yes' and 'no'. Instead, reframing them as 'negotiable' and 'non-negotiable' leaves more room for you to make decisions at a later date.

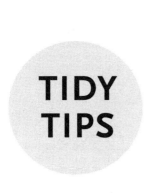

TIDY
TIPS

If there has been a traumatic ending to a life or a relationship, the process of decluttering and organising any space that is undergoing change will ultimately help you to let go.

Sometimes, we get thrown into situations and have no idea where to start. If that happens to you, always start by reducing things that are less sentimental and keeping the things that mean something – save these to go through another day. These items are the 'non-negotiables'; for example, the special chair that your mum sat in every day. There may be one outfit that you remember seeing her wear time and again that you will treasure. It might be the smell of your dad's aftershave, so you save the bottle. But that's enough.

REHOMING

My mum has a sideboard which she has owned for ever, where she stores all her fine-dining plates. I remember it from childhood. My mum certainly doesn't entertain, but she still wants to keep that dinner set. So, when she dies, I will find it very difficult to get rid of the crockery – and the sideboard – because she kept them for so long and they are significant to her. Do I have room for a sideboard and a whole set of plates?

I think I'll try to find a home for them with someone I know because I will be thinking sentimentally about where they are going. If you have similar items to rehome, it's important that anything you have inherited goes to someone who will benefit from it and who will enjoy it.

ONE BOX

I try to teach people that if they're facing difficult situations where they have to make tough decisions, it's helpful to think about what they would keep if they only had *one* box. What would be the most special things?

Have conversations with your family about their future plans, right now. Unless you're aware of their wishes, one day down the line you're going to be faced with questions that you don't know the answers to. And that's where the uncertainty lies and confusion will set in. Even though these conversations are awkward, I would suggest you have them.

These discussions also help to encourage your parents and older relatives to think about decluttering themselves, to remove the objects that they don't need or use right now; perhaps even sell them and put that money towards enjoying themselves. The reality is that most of us are not going to be able to absorb all our family members' belongings into our own homes because there isn't enough room. That's why you should focus on specifics and imagine that single box which will hold one outfit and one bottle of aftershave.

Start those conversations with your parents and also work out what is important in your own house. When you think about your own death and specifically about the possessions you'd like to hand down, I'm sure there won't be two hundred items or a whole house-worth of belongings that you feel it's essential your family saves. Instead, you'll be able to narrow it down to one or two *truly valuable* things, whether that's financially or sentimentally. What would you pass on that would *really* mean something? If the answer is very little or even nothing, get rid of it, or make some money from it, if you can.

Prepare for the future

Bring your thoughts back to your house in the present day and consider all the things in your home that you aren't using *now*, and that you'd instruct your family to get rid of in the event of your death.

All those books that you've had for years? Donate them to the library so that you've got less to worry about right now. You'll have less to oragnise and more time to enjoy yourself.

As we get older, we don't want to be managing the same house that we did when we were 30, 40 or 50. We want fewer clothes to wash, fold or iron and fewer ornaments to dust. Surely you don't still want to have eight wardrobes of clothes to choose from? When you're older, a small curated collection of items – in any category – makes much more sense.

You're hopefully not working as much as you did, so make it easy for yourself and free up your time to enjoy yourself, and your precious space.

MOVING HOUSE

You have decided that the best way to change your space is to physically move to another house. This will give you the opportunity for a fresh start and you can really look at how the new space will work for you. Before you plan where to put your furniture and what storage you might need, I've put together an essential checklist of things to consider when you're planning on moving house:

1. Declutter your existing possessions first.

2. Look at the floorplans of your new home and compare room sizes and storage options. Count the cupboards in your current and future kitchen. Does this home give you effective storage? If not, what are you planning to do?

3. What will you gain in your new space?

4. What have you lost?

5. What can be improved?

6. What room matters the most?

7. What did your last home lack?

8. What was the bugbear that you don't want to repeat?

Making a smooth transition into your new space starts with a little organisation, before you even begin to pack up your old house. On your new floorplan, write down what purpose you're assigning to each room and then add a list of what possessions should go in each. As you pack up your house, declutter as much as you can, so you're not taking anything broken or unused into the new space. Pre-plan and purchase any new storage you need, then pack with that storage in mind.

Always keep one box with you, containing essential items that you will need when you arrive (think: kettle, tea, coffee, milk, sugar, laptop and passports). Think of packing for a long weekend: pack a washbag, underwear and a change of clothes, along with children's school uniforms. You'll be able to live quite comfortably from your suitcase for a couple of days and won't have to rush around looking for socks when you arrive! Always unpack the important rooms first – usually that's the kitchen and bedrooms.

SEASONAL PLANNER

Autumn

As the leaves fall from the trees, it's a time of release. With the change in seasons comes the urge to switch our homes up again. It's autumn and that means kids heading back to school and families shifting back into the house after a summer spent outside. Make sure you're getting involved in this season's 7-Day Challenge (page 186), as it's so important to refresh your space every few months.

Autumn is a time to start looking inwards again.

The big change I notice in autumn is the way that I feel about my free time. I always feel that I tumble through summer, because there is so much going on! There's holidays and outings, and if you have children they need entertaining for many weeks. When you're spending so much time outside, you don't really have the opportunity to focus much on what's going on *inside* your house. Autumn is a time to start looking inwards again. It's almost like you're entering a lockdown phase! It's natural to be focused on your home because you're going out less.

Autumn is a great time to think about renovating and updating. You're also likely to start thinking about the holiday season, so don't try to fit in TOO many physical interior jobs. Work out the tasks that absolutely need to be done before the really dark days settle in.

Inside your home, the main area to tackle – and the most obvious one to get involved in at this time of year – is the bedroom and changing over your wardrobe. Autumn is the perfect season for a wardrobe cleanse. The September issues of fashion magazines are always the biggest month of the year (it's also my favourite season for fashion – I love wearing boots, cosy jumpers and cardigans). It's the time when you put away your summer clothes, sandals and swimwear, as it's unlikely you'll be needing them for the next few months!

BIG SPACE 1: BEDROOM AND WARDROBES

Questions to ask yourself before you start:

> Does it feel cluttered? We want to turn that around so it feels calm.

> Does the furniture need to be moved? Is there enough storage – wardrobe, drawers, underbed storage?

> Is there too much of anything – or too little? Do you have enough clothes hangers or drawer dividers?

Sofa love

Give your sofa a deep clean because you know you're going to be spending lots of time on it in the coming months.

> How are the clothes organised – do they work as they currently are?

> Can drawer items be hung, or hanging items be folded?

> Are there any random things that don't belong in the bedroom? Where can you move them to?

> How can you improve the aesthetic of the drawers and wardrobe?

> How can you ensure everything is accessible?

> How can you create a sanctuary so the bedroom becomes inviting?

1. Now, as always, clear everything out of the room first.

2. Consider whether you need to move any furniture around to make the room flow better. Can

you add any more storage (such as underbed drawers or boxes) to make things easier and give you more options?

3. Give the room a good clean and freshen it up.

4. Once your structure is in place, tackle the contents of your wardrobe and drawers...

WARDROBE

Go through your old summer clothes before you pack them away. Repair them or give any items that you didn't wear to charity. The chances are, if you didn't wear it this summer, you won't wear it again. I tend to wear on repeat the items that I really love and while I might add a few new things each season, it's worth checking what you are keeping before you store anything away. Group the clothes into sections (T-shirts, dresses, shorts, swimwear, etc.) and store them in small vacuum bags – one for each type of clothing. Label the bags and you will have no problem finding the things you need again when the next season rolls around.

If you already have your colder weather clothes in storage, get them out and check them over for damage. If not, just make sure you are putting the correct season's clothes back into your wardrobe and drawers. Ensure all your items are grouped and then put everything back in sections (just as you have done with your summer clothes). Keep shirts, winter dresses, skirts, trousers and jeans in separate places. This will make it so much easier when you're getting dressed.

You can hang lightweight knitwear, but heavy knits need to be folded. I always recommend narrow velvet hangers. They look neat but also take up minimal space. A jewellery box is always a good idea to stop precious and delicate pieces becoming tangled. Shoes and boots can be stored well on open shelving or a bookshelf, but always make sure what you are planning to use works for your needs.

Remember that while you're going to be snuggling up in cosy knitwear, it's good to keep one eye on the incoming party season, too. This year, could you think about hiring or borrowing special-occasion outfits instead of buying them? Renting clothing keeps your spending down, reduces the number of clothes you

Capsule wardrobe

Instead of buying 10 new items, can you build a capsule wardrobe with 10 items you already own?

Capsule wardrobes are a great idea, as they include a few essential pieces that all go with each other. This allows you to have outfits that always work, whatever the occasion. These trans-seasonal pieces will work hard across the year with just a few seasonal additions:

> Blazer (or other smart jacket)

> Casual jacket (like a bomber, biker or shacket)

> Versatile dress (choose a hard-working dress that will take you from the school run to cocktails with just a change of accessories)

> Casual weekend dress in denim or twill

> Smart trousers (you can make these look formal or casual, depending on your accessories)

> Statement skirt (choose something that feels special but that you can still dress down)

> Shirt or blouse (make sure your top options all go, colour-wise, with your bottoms)

> Plain T-shirt

> Jumper

> Jeans (choose a style that suits your shape and your lifestyle)

have that only get a rare outing and is better for the environment, too. You do *not* need to buy 10 new items a month.

A summer filled with day trips and holidays can be expensive, so autumn is a chance to reframe your thinking and your spending patterns.

DOLLY DASH 1

Linen cupboard

Autumn is the time to change your bedding and blankets. You're making sure everything around you feels lovely, cosy and welcoming. Doing a Dolly Dash on your towels and linen cupboard is a very quick way to make your home feel aligned to the seasons.

Check that your sheets, pillows and duvets are all in good condition. Do you need to switch over to brushed cotton bedding instead of lightweight fabrics? Launder and put away summer-weight duvets and bring out winter ones.

Are your towels warm and fluffy? In summer, I don't mind what my towels are like, but in autumn I crave thick towels that are going to dry me quickly to keep me warm.

Make time to go through your blankets and throws – give them a freshen up in the wash before you pop them back on your sofa, all nicely folded. That way, when you're ready to snuggle up in your living room, the blankets will smell lovely and feel fluffy, too. It also makes sense to think of textures and colours that are comforting and warming, so think about what you could swap around for the season.

BIG SPACE 2:
THE LOFT

Lofts can be a tricky space to access, so I always recommend organising as much stuff while you are physically *in* the loft as you can, as it can be awkward to bring everything down. (Clothes are an exception, as you can sort through them quite easily downstairs. Likewise, photos and albums are also small enough to bring down. Going through old photos makes a lovely project that you can tackle as a family, over a longer period of time.)

Start by moving everything to one side of the loft, so you have a blank space on the other side and can start creating sections. As with any other space, go through all your possessions and group them together. Get rid of duplicates, anything broken or damaged that you know you will no longer use, and make a plan to donate or recycle these quickly, so they don't take up valuable space in your house.

Use the beams of the loft as helpful section dividers to begin with.

DOLLY DASH 2

Kids' things

Autumn is another good time to look at your children's things. Kids go through periods of change so much faster than adults. Every season brings major developments for them as they grow.

Autumn is the start of a new school year – they'll be reading new books and studying different materials. They'll be ready for new clothes or uniform (again!), so keep an eye on their wardrobes – clearing out the old summer clothes and those that no longer fit. Declutter books that are too young for their reading age, colouring books that are filled in and toys that have been outgrown.

You could allocate one section to travel, one for Christmas, one for Halloween, one for camping, and so on.

The key to organising your loft is to put everything into labelled containers, so it's easy to find what you need rather than having a mass of black bags and no idea what's inside them.

With suitcases, always put smaller cases inside bigger cases to save space. Small weekend bags and trolleys can easily fit inside larger ones.

When it's time to decide what sections go where, use the areas closest to the hatch for things you will need to access more often, and the rear of the loft for those that will be least used. Items like suitcases, camping kit and seasonal celebration boxes for Christmas, Halloween and Easter may be towards the front of the loft, while memorabilia can live at the back.

Save the loft for autumn

I have cleaned out many lofts in mid-summer and they get hot! Autumn is the ideal time to tackle this area.

LIFE LESSON

Through my work I've seen that the biggest changes that need to be made in the home are often undertaken by blended families. Yet I've noticed with *all* the families that I've worked with that people don't use their space effectively. The biggest change my clients have to make is actually realising how to make the most of the space they have and facilitating this.

Frequently, people get thrown into a new space or a situation where they have to share their space, but don't make any fundamental changes to the shape of rooms, the layout of furniture or the way that the home flows. And this puts strain on the family relationships. Often, rooms will remain exactly the same as they were before the change and no one has managed to adapt to the new situation.

When I start on a house declutter, I always analyse why the space isn't working for that family and try to work out what they are doing wrong. Nine times out of ten, the spaces aren't working because they simply haven't been properly considered. The family tends to throw themselves into the house and get on with living without taking a step back and asking:

'Are we making the most of this space now our situation has changed?'

I've also seen this problem in military families, or those who need to move often. Some people can become so attached to their possessions it becomes debilitating, because 'things' are all they have.

These peripatetic families can never become attached to a house because they're only living there for a couple of years before they need to move again; therefore possessions become the only thing that the family can connect to. Yet I've seen so many times that too many belongings can end up swamping a family.

I worked with one family who had finally moved into their forever home and were happy, at last. They had changed their physical space, but it had the added effect that they now felt they could get rid of many of their possessions because they had a connection with their home, at last. This signalled a major change – to the benefit of everyone in the household.

The essence of this chapter is that change in your life *has* to mean changing your attitude in order to change your space. Otherwise you will suffer. When *nothing* changes in your physical space but *everything* is changing in your life, you will be out of balance. Always remember to frequently question what the people in your house really need and ensure that the space works for everyone.

Change in your life has to mean changing your attitude in order to change your space.

PART FOUR

ACCEPT

your situation

ACCEPT (verb), 1: to believe or come to recognise a proposition as valid or correct; **2:** to consider someone or something as satisfactory.

MY STORY

Chaos had such an impact on my life growing up, as well as my mum and dad's lives. I truly believe the cause of my mum's mental health struggles was the fact that they both worked so hard. They worked every single hour of the day as chartered accountants and it took over their marriage. It had a detrimental effect on me because they didn't come to school to collect me – I had to walk to the local supermarket, which didn't close until 8pm, to wait for them there.

Strangely, this minimart was where my organisation journey began, aged 10. It was a safe place for me to wait, so to pass the time I would rearrange the shelves, help people pack their shopping and tidy up the aisles.

From those earliest days, I could see the difference that bringing order to a space can make to your mood and your mental health.

It was also around this time that I came to realise my parents were workaholics and I knew that the chaos, unrest and clutter in their house was never going to change. My parents wanted to give me the best life possible, but it was clear that the house was never going to be their priority. Somehow I knew that I had to accept that situation – it was just the way they were.

When I was younger, I didn't notice the chaos so much, but as I got older and spent more time in my own room, I realised that I could have control over the space I was in. Likewise, as my mum spent more time in hospital (and I headed into my tweens and early teens), I was naturally able to take control over the rest of the house. From my early acceptance of the fact that I couldn't change anything, beyond keeping my own bedroom tidy, I came to understand that if I wanted the rest of the space to change, *I* was the one who had to do it, not my parents. I think for many of us, once we realise that *we* have to be the one to make the change and not anyone else, that's where the power shift begins and you can start to declutter your life.

If you are stuck in a rut with your home or fed up with how it functions, get involved in sorting it out! If you are desperate to gain back some control and want to live a more organised, clearer and calmer life, you need to accept that you must change it.

Accept that the reason that your home has so much stuff in it is *you*. The reason that your kids' toys are taking over every inch of your home is because *you* are buying them (you know I'm also guiltily sighing at this!).

The reason your wardrobe is overflowing with fast fashion (yet you still have nothing to wear) is *you*.

'Have nothing in your house that you do not know to be useful or believe to be beautiful.'

William Morris

You really need to love every piece in your wardrobe, every item in your home, otherwise why on earth do you have it? Seriously, why?! If it's not something that makes your face hurt because you can't stop smiling when you wear it, it doesn't belong in your wardrobe. The same applies to home accessories. Stop overbuying toys for the kids. Stop overbuying snacks. Stop stocking up on paper towels. You don't need it all.

Slow it right down. Accept that you can live with less.

Are you ready to admit that change is the only thing you need to commit to in your life?

KEY LIFE CHANGE

Decluttering is about motivating yourself to really want that change. And you need to keep asking, 'How much do I want it?' because nothing is going to happen without you and your willpower. I won't hide that it can be hard to commit to the whole process, so you have to be in the right frame of mind to tackle it properly. You really do need to be ready and make sure you have the right tools and support in place in order to do anything big like making a difference in your home.

Unfortunately, humans are not programmed to enjoy change. It's in our nature to fear it, to dread it. But when you get through a period of change, life can often be so much better. It's like living healthily and taking control of your diet. We all know that when you eat better, stop drinking wine every night of the week, move away from a processed, high-sugar diet and do some exercise, you'll feel better. But when you don't *want* to cut back on the wine, the sugar and the late-night snacks, it's because you're not really ready for that change. When you do decide that you're ready to stick to it, you will smash your goals.

I always remind my clients that the sooner they can realise the benefits of change and envision how much their life will transform, the better their lives will be. That's when you'll be ready to go for it!

'Life is too complicated not to be orderly.'

Martha Stewart

SCENARIO: DIVORCE

When you are dealing with divorce and potentially dividing up your home, accept that you have to think about the things that are going to make you feel better, rather than dwell on the things of the past. Will you feel better by arguing over pieces of furniture? Or would you rather be sat on a bare floor with nothing and build yourself up again? Work out what is taking up more of your energy. Sometimes you will realise that you are wasting time and energy by arguing over something as trivial as furniture. You may have put money into every purchase you made together, but could you wait six months and then buy that piece of furniture (or something you love even more) for yourself?

Change can be a golden opportunity for a fresh start. One door has closed but another one has opened. Please keep reminding yourself of the vision you have for your future and remember that this point in the journey is only temporary – a short-term situation. If you keep considering where you were before this and the place where you want to be, it will make even the most awful 'now' worth it.

Accepting that items you once owned don't necessarily serve you any more, and that it's no longer beneficial for you to be living among them, is also a really helpful step in the process.

I have enough and that is everything.

SCENARIO: HAVING A BABY

When you're having a baby, it's inevitable that change will occur. It's likely that you have accepted that there will be sleepless nights and fewer nights out, but what you might not have realised is how a new baby will affect your entire home. Do you have room for all the extra *stuff* that accompanies a baby? Will you have to move your home office into the living room to make way for a nursery? How will that affect your job? Dealing with these day-to-day situations can impact your relationship, mental health and space. I believe that the best way to get to a place of acceptance is by planning how these physical changes will affect your house and considering how that will make you feel from day to day.

If you can plan for changes to your space, you'll be in a much better place, because it's only when you DON'T plan for change that you end up in disarray.

I recommend you start to think about allocating a cupboard for the baby in the kitchen, clearing out wardrobe space and considering whether you will be storing a pram in your hall (making it narrower and perhaps meaning you have to lose a piece of furniture). Plan ahead for what happens when you move the baby into their own room (or whether they are sharing with a sibling). This will help you balance the relationships with everyone in the household, so you can *all* accept how things will change at home.

SCENARIO: BEREAVEMENT

Anyone who has lost a loved one will realise that grief doesn't end, it just changes shape as time goes on. For some people, that shape doesn't necessarily get smaller. I've seen that accepting that you have to live without a loved one – that your life will never be the same – can be incredibly hard.

Everyone has their own reaction to grief. You have to take it at your own pace.

There is no right or wrong way to be when you are grieving, but slowly learning to adjust to this new situation will help you accept the fact that this loss will remain with you for ever.

I want to share the suggestion that you may be able to reach a point of acceptance more easily if you transfer your loss onto something physical. By acknowledging that the person you loved is no longer there, but an object that they loved (and that you can enjoy) *is* still present is often a great comfort. Perhaps they loved a particular flower, or there's a scent that reminds you of them. Planting those flowers in your garden or a special place, or bringing them into your home, is a lovely way to hold on to special memories of happier times.

Perhaps there was a vase that your granny loved, or maybe you can bring a special picture into your space. These objects will bring you joy every time you look at them,

Preparing for a baby together

This is one for both you and your partner to get involved in. Each write down five things you think need to change in your space before the baby arrives.

Discuss them and then make a priority plan for how you will implement those changes.

Next, both write down the top three things that you *don't* want to change (maybe that's having a quiet WFH space or getting a full night's sleep when you're working). Again, discuss how you can make those priorities a reality. Consider starting a sleep rota, for instance.

Thinking ahead and planning around the finer details, which sometimes get overlooked, will allow you all to accept the wonderful changes that are coming your way.

because you'll be reminded of your loved one. Use the memories you have and turn them into something positive. By cherishing these things, you can keep your memories alive. When we lose someone, we don't have to shed ourselves of everything they owned and start afresh. Holding on to a few things that make you feel happy will bring you joy and help you reach a place of acceptance.

Naturally, for some people, it's still easier not to look at items that remind them of their loss. It's up to you to decide what you feel ready to deal with, but I have seen that when you have something dear to you in a prominent place, the pain does ease.

You will never get rid of the grief, but one day you will get to a point where you can accept it and live with it as part of your everyday existence.

Holding on to a few things that make you feel happy will bring you joy and help you reach a place of acceptance.

THE BIG PICTURE

It's so important to frequently revisit how you feel about your rooms, your space and your home. How would you like them to be? Consider what they look like right now.

There is a start, a middle and an end for every decluttering journey.

At the beginning, you may be faced with a chaotic situation. Maybe it's a spare room where you can't see the floor, or a cupboard that has hundreds of items toppling out every time you try to open it. That's the scenario *before* you start to declutter. To move on from this point, you have to make a change. Think about what you need to do to make the space work better, or how can you make it more beneficial to your family. Making that conscious decision to begin is the first step in the process. The middle part is *during* the decluttering process, when you are clearing the room, emptying that cupboard, editing and removing unwanted items from your space. It can feel like a huge task, but remember you've already made progress. When you reach the point where you are faced with a blank space and you can decide what goes back (tightly edited and organised, of course), you're on the home stretch! Eventually, you will reach the end point where your room is reset. Time to celebrate! But also take a moment to think about the place this journey has taken you to – the 'after'.

My feeling is that the end scenario is never fully 'the end'.

Document how far you've come

Work out how far away your current situation is from your vision. Visualise the end – the 'after' – of your decluttering journey and think about how you would describe your feelings in that new space.

That feeling of completion is the moment when you should feel proud of what you've done, for what you have achieved. It's a great idea to make notes as you progress on your journey.

Take a 'before' photograph, a 'during', then an 'after'. Look back and see how far you've come. Acknowledge the feelings you had in the early days of your journey, then compare them to how you are feeling right now, now you've done it.

It's good to have a reminder of where you came from. The 'after' is always the most exhilarating point, because you will be free from whatever held you back in your home.

Keep going back to that space, reminding yourself of the calm and ease you feel in your house when it's decluttered, and this will help you maintain control of your home.

EMBRACE THE JOURNEY

Often we hang on to the negatives and focus on the bad points of our lives. I regularly show clients before-and-after pictures to remind them of how far they've come. It's easy to be in the now and to forget the place you came from. In my personal experience, I often forget that I lived very well for most of my life. I focus on my mum's illness, how hard it was for her, and how that impacted me. But actually, my life was never bad. I went to private school until I was seven. I lived on a beautiful road surrounded by lovely neighbours, and we had lots of friends and family. Maybe the reason I hang on to the negatives is because my mum is now living at the bottom of my garden, so I have a constant reminder. If she was out of sight, maybe she would be out of mind. But I want you to remember the whole process of your decluttering journey – the process of change.

I want you to think about how that journey has affected you in the past and how it's affecting you now.

Change isn't easy – it's an evolving process, but it's essential that you appreciate all the places you've travelled through to get here. This will help you to appreciate how you're going to get on with life again and accept whatever situation you are in.

Do something today that your future self will thank you for.

The place to aim for is the other side of the process, when you can enjoy the results and spend your time in a clean, calm and decluttered space. When you can light some lovely smelling candles and have plumped-up cushions to relax on. That vision of future comfort will help you balance out your fear of change. Right now, you might be dealing with the negative attachment you have to items that came from a difficult time. If you're still trying to hold on to those items, perhaps it's time to move them out of your life.

'To accomplish great things, we must not only act, but also dream; not only plan, but also believe.'

Anatole France

Vision is one of the most important elements of this process, but change can only happen with you. Think back to the beginning of your journey and the start of this book when you were feeling negative and struggling with your home. I hope you can see that you can compartmentalise the issues that were troubling you in each section of your life. Which segment of this book affected you the most? How are you feeling now? I'm hoping you now have a vision and a plan and can move forward, that you understand *why* you need to do the tasks, as well as *how* to do them.

It's up to you now. *You* need to make sure that change happens. You *can* implement that change.

Change starts with you and it ends with you.

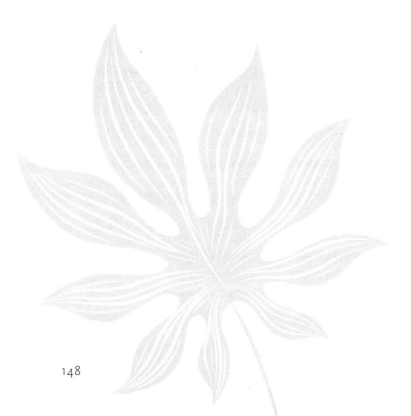

LOOK AFTER YOURSELF

'With organisation comes empowerment.'

Lynda Peterson

I wouldn't be here, telling my story and sharing my advice, if it wasn't for my mum and dad coming to Sri Lanka and bringing me back to England. When I've gone through some of the hardest, toughest times in my life, I take a step back and remember to write down the things that I *do* have, and this is a method I'd suggest you consider too.

Make a list of things you are grateful for. It's so easy to focus on the bad things in life – but there are always positives. As well as doing this exercise at the toughest points in your life, it's a good idea to get into the habit of being grateful every week, if you can, or at least every month.

Over the course of the chapters in this book, we have focused on your house, your life and the negatives within them, but it's important to keep in mind the good things too. We all deal with so many things throughout our lives. You might be forgetting that you were brave enough to leave a bad relationship or a really horrible marriage. That's a positive. You may be combining two families together and starting an amazing new chapter in your life. There are difficulties but it comes from a place of love, which is amazing. You may have lost a deeply beloved relative, but what will never leave you are the lessons that you learned from them and the time that you spent together.

WELLBEING BENEFITS

When you have realised that change has to happen and you have accepted it, it makes any further decisions easier to deal with. If you're struggling with a tricky choice and you're battling against a set of difficult circumstances, you're constantly challenging yourself. Once you open your mind to the change and engage with any support that you need, decisions will become easier. Looking objectively at your situation will help you acknowledge and value what you have and may also help you realise that that very same situation may not be serving you right now. There comes a point where you will be able to let go and accept the change and then everything will become clear.

I have accepted that my mum is now living at the end of my garden. It's vital that you too learn to accept the situation you may have found yourself in. I encourage you to think about how you can make the best of it, even when it seems like a bad situation or one that you didn't want. I have found that changing your mindset to one of acceptance is key to long-term happiness and wellbeing.

Accept that this new situation, this new way of living, this new environment or set-up is here right now and is your reality. It's truly your choice whether you continue to battle the situation, or whether you accept it and learn work-arounds to make the most of it. This approach of acceptance will bring so many benefits to you, your family and whoever the change is currently affecting.

Once you've reached the point of acceptance and you've realised all the good things that you *do* have, then you will be able to properly appreciate the situation. This will ultimately allow you to move on to happier times.

Approaching change

In your notebook, write down five things that are positive in your life.

Then, think of five things that are negative – the situations and things you want to change. Remember that, although they might be negative, *you* have the power to change them. Ultimately, you're in control.

Finally, write down five things that you aren't happy with, that you *can't* change and need to learn to accept. Think deeper on those last five points. Is there room for *any* movement?

There are many situations you *can't* change, but perhaps, if you try, you will find a way to frame them differently. You could turn your negatives into positives if you learn to accept them.

I want to remind you of where we've journeyed in this book. Yes, you may have lost someone. Yes, your marriage may have broken down. Yes, I was adopted. Yes, my mum suffers with her mental health. But sometimes the toughest things to deal with are the things we learn from the most. We can be grateful for this.

Change is inevitable. Accept that it happens.

You know by now that change itself is often something you can't control, but taking charge of how you deal with it and your destructive habits is in your power and means you are making a positive step towards the future.

I know you don't enjoy it (none of us do!), but you need to remain grateful in the long run for the opportunities change presents and remember all the positives you have experienced.

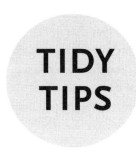

TIDY TIPS

GIVE YOURSELF TIME

Looking back on everything I've experienced in my life, I've realised the importance of both time and responsibility. These two things are constantly changing as our lives move on. Right now, I live in a home with three generations of family. The childhood that Charley and I can give Nelly is totally different from my own but that doesn't mean that I wish my own experience was different. I truly believe I wouldn't be here now if Mum hadn't been ill. I learned how to be responsible from an early age and then, over time, those early responsibilities affected my whole outlook on life, which led me to my organising mission. I have learnt to embrace the good and the bad and take on every challenge, accepting the lessons from each experience I've gone through.

Time is key to accepting change – learning to allow new situations to become part of your life takes investment. Whether you have lost a loved one, are affected by illness or are welcoming a new member to your household, it's important to remember not to make changes too quickly.

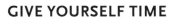

Our lives can change in a heartbeat and we need to give ourselves enough time to adjust.

The more ordered and organised I am, the easier my life is – I've learnt to adapt, share, change and, last but not least, to accept. Remember, you can control your response to what happens to you (both emotionally and in your environment) but you can't control the actions of others.

5 WAYS TO PRACTISE ACCEPTANCE

In the same way I believe it's important to practise gratitude, I also think it's essential to practise acceptance.

Learning to accept and embrace change is so important for your wellbeing, both now and in the future.

Follow these 5 Ps – they can be applied to both your emotional self and your physical space.

1. **Process** – Give yourself enough time to accept changes; don't make any big changes too quickly.

2. **Plan** – Make sure you assess where you are at and decide what you need to do first, in a considered manner.

3. **Prepare** – Ease your way into the process and make small, manageable changes first.

4. **Purpose** – Remember, you can control how you decide to look forwards. Think about what you want your future to look like, then work towards making those changes.

5. **Possibility** – Every change opens a door to new possibilities. If you look beyond your current horizon, perhaps you'll discover bigger, even more positive changes ahead.

Beyond inner acceptance, I suggest you take action and re-frame your situation by taking practical steps to organise your home. Keep your vision of happier times at the front of your mind so you can focus on the physical changes. You'll be able to take the steps needed to realise them with ease.

PLANNING AND DOING

When you are ready to tackle your home following a big change, use the same process you'd apply when approaching any decluttering: always start by making time to consider what needs to happen. Get yourself a mug of something and sit down with your notebook to properly plan and visualise the result.

HOW TO CREATE A TIMELINE FOR MAKING CHANGE

When you start to schedule decluttering tasks, it's important to dedicate enough time to each element. You can easily lose motivation if you feel the process isn't moving as fast as you would like. Realistically considering how much time you will need – and writing that in your timeline – is crucial.

Of course, there are 15-minute Dolly Dashes that you can undertake, but thinking your kitchen will only take a couple of hours to sort out (when it's been untouched since you moved in 15 years ago) will only lead to setbacks, demotivation and disappointment when you run out of time or become overwhelmed.

Look at your diary and decide what windows of time you can allocate to making changes, then divide those blocks into big, medium or smaller sessions that realistically fit into your timeline. Stick to those slots in the same way you would if it was a doctor's appointment or meeting a friend.

Setting aside a dedicated thinking space will give you valuable time to get ready for the changes in your home. When you think through what needs to happen, work your way back from the finished scenario. I recommend you schedule any changes over a period of time that has a clear start – and end – point to keep you motivated.

If you feel stuck during this process, remind yourself of my 6 Golden Rules of Decluttering (page 18): Assess; Clear; Group; Categorise; Store; Label. These steps, when done in order, will help you tidy any area of your home.

STAY MOTIVATED

It's worth repeating, decluttering is not a 'one and done' solution.

You constantly have to come back and keep an eye on every area of your home so you don't revert to bad habits, even if you have reached a point of acceptance.

This is why I recommend you use the 7-day seasonal challenges or the 30-day challenges in the next chapter of this book as an easy way to reset. Set these as future goals (and stick to them) and you will find it so much easier to continue to live with, and accept your new situation.

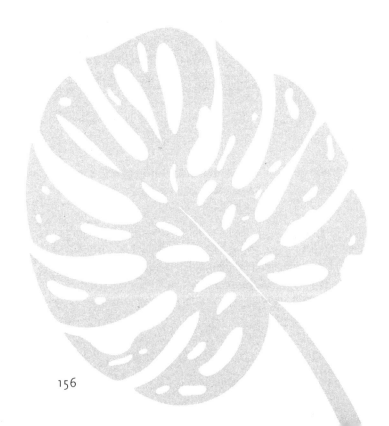

SEASONAL PLANNER

Winter

Winter is the time when we hibernate. While you're inside all the time, it makes sense to declutter the rooms you spend the most time in. There are also many opportunities to decorate our homes in winter – Halloween, Christmas – so it's particularly important that you keep on top of the organisation so your homes are ready to bedeck and you're ready to entertain. There are always people popping in and out, particularly during December, and you want to be ready to welcome your friends and family into the warm. You can't get festive on top of clutter!

Winter is also a time to look after yourself. It's cold and flu season, so make sure your medicine cupboard is fully stocked. When did you last go through your medicines and check everything is still in date? Likewise, when did you check that the kids' wellies still fit? Have you unpacked your winter coats, hats, scarves and gloves ready for the inclement weather? Are you prepared for the season ahead? Stock up on logs for your fireplace, if you have one, and check you have enough supplies for the season.

I find that winter is the best time to start going through your crockery, cutlery and glasses in preparation for events ahead. Party season is coming, so make sure your house is ready! Your bedding needs to be in the best condition too, as you'll definitely be spending more time cosying up. When it's cold outside, you will want to be swaddled in warm, good-quality fabrics.

Once you've got the practicalities sorted, you can enjoy all the fun elements of the season, whether that's reading a book by the fire or entertaining!

BIG SPACE 1: KITCHEN

How to create a kitchen that flows:

> Set aside 6–8 hours to tackle this.

> Empty the entire contents of the kitchen into the largest, clearest space next to the kitchen (don't just empty the cupboards onto the worktops – you will feel claustrophobic and not be able to organise efficiently). You need to be able to work in a blank space.

> Start to group everything into categories: baking, tins, Tupperware, pots and pans, glassware, ceramics (plates, bowls, mugs), cutlery.

> Next tackle food: pasta, pulses, tinned food, snacks. Go through and discard anything out of date or broken.

> Look it all over and decide what you need and what you don't.

> Do you need multiples of things? When did you use it last? Is it sentimental? Do you have a valid financial reason for keeping something? Make a pile of things you are going to get rid of.

> The next crucial step is to put everything into containers. The reason we use baskets, crates or containers is not just to keep things looking neat, it's to control the amount of each thing we own. Unlike so many organisers, who just decant things into matching jars because it looks pretty, I want you to realise that the containers are there to give you a guideline as to what you need to own and what quantity of it fits into your space. Unless you can clearly see into them, labelling the containers will make sure you don't forget what is inside each one. If you can't label the containers, can you label the shelves instead?

> Now look at the structure of the kitchen. Can you move the position of shelves within cupboards? Can you add shelves? Could you add cutlery organisers or drawer dividers? When you've got the structure sorted, you can start to move items back in.

> Give each shelf, drawer and cupboard a purpose. Things you access daily should be lower down; things you rarely use can be stored higher up. Try not to keep things you very rarely use in your main kitchen.

> Start moving items back into their new homes in their groups. Keeping like-for-like items together is key to a calm, organised aesthetic.

> Try not to mix glass with ceramics.

DOLLY DASH 1

Fridge/freezer

At this time of year, you will want to have as much space in your fridge and freezer as possible, especially if you're entertaining or want to store Christmas leftovers! Get your fridge and freezer in the best shape possible by completely emptying them and thoroughly cleaning every shelf and drawer.

Get rid of anything out of date, then group all the foods that you have removed into sections. Put them into containers so you can clearly see what you've got. This will stop you from overbuying in future and potentially wasting food.

Now you can put the containers back in an organised manner. You could try using stacking containers to save space but don't forget you can adjust the shelf heights in your appliance to make the space work for you. I always label each shelf and container so I know where everything should go. Each drawer or shelf should have a clear purpose to help you stay tidy.

> Try not to mix Tupperware with pots and pans.

> Remember to donate or recycle anything you don't need.

> Cleaning your kitchen is obviously a really important exercise to help you practise good food hygiene, but it's also really beneficial to your mental health, to know your kitchen is clean, tidy and hygienic. .

BIG SPACE 2: BATHROOM

> Allow 2–3 hours to clear your bathroom.

> Clear all products from the windowsills and the sides of your bath and shower. Empty the cupboards, cabinets and any storage units.

> When empty, thoroughly clean the entire space.

> Now start to go through your products. Reduce what you don't need and get rid of duplicates. Are there products you bought to test that didn't work for you? Can you donate anything to a beauty bank? Only keep the items that you use every day.

> When you've gone through everything, group the remaining items by category. Create a section for skincare, dental, personal hygiene, haircare, body, bath products, fake tan, etc.

> Give each shelf in your bathroom a clear purpose. If you have only a few shelves, divide them into two, so each half has a distinct purpose.

> Consider whether any items (make-up, for example) can go into the bedroom, rather than being kept in the bathroom, to free up more space.

> Work out whether you need an extra storage unit or perhaps another shelf.

> The goal is for your bathroom to feel light, relaxing and inviting and not be a space cluttered with products that don't get used.

> Make sure that the windowsills are clear. You want as much light in the space as possible, so try not to fill the windowsill with clutter and products that will block the light.

DOLLY DASH 2

Make-up bag

If you're wearing more make-up in winter, as you socialise more, this is the ideal time to Dolly Dash your make-up bag.

You should only keep the products that you use every day in your make-up bag. If you have excess items, store them in a shoebox, perhaps tucked under your bed.

Old make-up can harbour bacteria and bugs that you keep putting back on your face (which can lead to infections), so check that everything you're using is still in date. Mascara and eyeliner need to be replaced after three months; concealer, cream blush, eyeshadow and lip gloss last for one year; powder blush and lipstick can last for two years.

Clean out your make-up bag and then thoroughly wash all your brushes with a gentle shampoo, before letting them dry on a towel. Sharpen your eye and lip pencils and wipe the lids, rims and sides of your products to remove any excess.

Giving everything a good clean, so it all feels fresh, will make putting your make-up on feel joyful.

LIFE LESSON

The biggest lesson you can learn from this book, from watching my Instagram or seeing me on TV, over and above the importance of the process of decluttering, is acknowledging that you need to *look* at a space to change that space.

SEE the problems and ACCEPT that they are problems, then resolve to CHANGE them.

Changing your space is one of the most important things that you can do.

So often we set up our homes on day one of moving in and don't think about the actual space. We don't take the time to look around and ask, 'How is this best going to work for us?' Sometimes we just empty stuff into a room and that's it! The biggest lesson you can learn from any type of decluttering or organisation process is that you need to effectively change the space first.

Always imagine your space as empty, then plan what you want it to be. The next step is to make it happen.

In order to do that, you have to start from the beginning and that means returning it to a blank canvas. You can now reinvent that area – you just need to rethink it. Do that and then the space will work better for you – it will be more effective.

So many people try to change a space while their items are still in it. But what I've learned from past experience – and what I want you to take away from this book – is that when a space is empty, it's easier to reimagine it.

In my decluttering work, I see kitchens as a prime example of where people don't like change and can struggle to accept it is needed. They become so used to the way the kitchen flows and, even if it doesn't really flow well, it can feel like the norm. When families have lived among chaos for so long, they come to accept it. Yet, when I change it for them, when I turn it around, they instantly recognise how beneficial – how needed – the change was.

I'm often booked for jobs and *still* have to convince the homeowners that my expertise in changing their house is going to benefit them. It can take a few hours, but even as I'm working I can see from the way their faces brighten that they realise how beneficial my changes will be. By the end of the job, they have accepted that this is the best thing they could have done and I can see a physical change in their whole body.

PART FIVE

CHALLENGE
yourself

I believe it's essential to keep on top of your belongings at all times. As a nation, we are constantly spending money. We buy new things every single day. We shop for food, we're constantly searching online for clothes, books, household items. We share occasions throughout the year, whether it's birthdays, anniversaries or Christmas, which involve gifts and keepsakes. There are new things coming into our homes daily, sometimes several times a day, which is why it's crucial that you undertake the challenges I've outlined in this chapter, to allow you to really maintain your space.

These challenges will not only give you the opportunity to reset your house, but will help refresh your mindset.

There is a 30-day challenge that will reframe your thinking in a big way, along with four smaller 7-day exercises, which follow the seasons, to give you the opportunity for a regular clear-out.

Day 1 or
one day...
it's your
choice.

30 DAYS OF CHANGE CHALLENGE

However organised you are and however tidy you keep your home, I recommend everyone gets on board with this challenge, particularly as the seasons change and the way you live in your house shifts throughout the year. Completing this challenge isn't a quick fix – it's a daily commitment for a whole month – but this is going to change your entire mindset.

The idea originated from bloggers @theminimalists and you can find it online using the hashtags #minsgame or #minimalistchallenge. I do this challenge every month that has 30 days in it (so 4 months per year). Join in if you can, otherwise you could take up the challenge biannually, or once a year, if that's all you can manage. The idea is that over the course of 30 days you remove as much as you can from your house, starting with one item on day one and increasing the amount every day. On day 2 you'll remove 2 things, and so on... all the way to day 30 (when you lose 30 objects from your space!).

At the end of the challenge you will have removed at least 465 items from your home.

I want you to change the way you consume and consider what you are bringing into your home. Get ready for big ideas that will make a transformational impact on the way your home functions, for ever.

This could be the first day of you changing your life. I want you to think about how much you need to change. Think about how it will affect the way that your home functions and how it could improve your relationships with others, as well as the positive benefits for yourself. The more in control you are of your space, the better you'll feel.

Are you ready to begin?

DAY 1

Today, you will remove just one object from your home. As you are only removing a single thing, look for a large item that will make a big impact. Think: large appliances or bulky furniture that doesn't fit your space. Is there a kid's wardrobe that has been outgrown or an unused occasional chair that's become a dumping ground for clothes? If you can reuse something in another area of the home, that counts too! For example, could a chest of drawers go into the garage to be used as storage? The early days of this challenge will help you create physical space in your home, which will make a huge difference to your interior decor and act as motivation for the remaining days.

DAY 2

Remove two items from your home. While the numbers are low, keep looking for big items you can remove. What do you have in your home that you no longer need? What are the things that will free up the most space? Is there an outgrown pushchair that can be donated or an unused bike lurking in the hall that can be sold? What about a rocking horse or doll's house that is gathering dust? Take them out!

DAY 3

Today you need to remove three objects. Look through your kitchen cupboards to find gadgets and appliances you never use. Perhaps you have a pasta machine, bread maker, deep-fat fryer or slow cooker that never sees the light of day. Does your microwave even get used? Make sure everything is truly earning its place in your kitchen, whether it's stored on the side or hidden in a cupboard or drawer. Every day of this challenge is designed to make you think deeply about those items you have in your home but never use, that just sit there taking up valuable space!

WHERE WILL YOUR STUFF GO?

As you go through the next 30 days, it's important to decide where the things you clear out will go. Do you need somewhere to store the things you're going to recycle or donate? If you don't work out where you're going to be disposing of or donating your items, a sense of claustrophobia is going to set in, which might derail your decluttering challenge. Think about the waste problems we have globally and ask yourself, where will this stuff go?

Research is key. Investigate what local businesses will collect items from your house, or where there are drop-off points. Check your local Facebook or Freecycle network. There are companies out there who will buy all your DVDs and books from you. Local schools, animal shelters and refuge centres may take paper, towels, sheets and hygiene products. Supermarkets often have clothes-recycling banks and there are textile-recycling banks in several high-street stores. Make phone calls and get online to work out where you need to go next.

It will be hard work, but nothing worth doing comes easily. You may find yourself driving around doing numerous drop-offs (although there are plenty of companies that will pick up items from your doorstep). But, if you want to reclaim the space in your home and change your life, it's worth it. And remember: one person's trash is another's treasure.

DAY 4

If you can, always try to remove items from the area that affects you the most, early on in the process. That way, you'll see big results – fast. Once the hardest areas are done, the rest will feel easy in comparison. Today, I'd like you to look at your hallway. Bulky winter coats take up a lot of room, but do you have coats hanging up that you no longer wear? Or perhaps you're just not wearing them at the moment. If this is the case, you could pack them up and put them away until next winter. Sometimes decluttering doesn't mean getting rid of things entirely.

DAY 5

As we're working on small numbers, keep focused on removing the largest items from your home. Today I'd like you to look at your outside space, if you have some. You should definitely be considering lofts, garages and sheds during this challenge. I guarantee you'll find plenty of items you could dispose of. Do you have a lawn mower that doesn't work or a trampoline you could sell?

DAY 6

Today it's time to remove six items from your home. Whichever area you focus on, I suggest that vision is the single most important thing you need to change your space. You have realised that your home isn't working, but why? We've gone through likely issues with the space in previous chapters, but I advise you to imagine every room as a blank canvas. What would you change if you could? Are the wardrobes in the wrong place? Is it the desk or the bed? Then ask yourself: what is the item that ruins the room the most? Is it too many clothes? Paperwork? Too many books? Too many toys? How can you improve the storage in your home and make it work better for you?

Work out a way for each room to be more aesthetically pleasing as well as more functional. You can write a list of what you need to do to make your vision for a room to come to life, working backwards from your goal through to the starting point, before starting to action these ideas.

'A good system shortens the road to the goal.'

Ralph Waldo Emerson

DAY 7

Let's go through your Tupperware. Bring everything out onto the work surface. Make sure every bottom has a top that matches. If there are lone pieces that don't match, see if you can recycle them or repurpose them as storage in a chest of drawers. Once you have matched up each set of Tupperware, store them – with lids on – inside each other. Then consider what you can reduce. Are there boxes that are too small (or too big) that you can remove, because you never use them or they're duplicates?

DAY 8

Have you been through your shoes recently? Are there any you're definitely not going to wear again that you can donate to charity or sell? If you live with others, can you go through their shoes, too? The goal is to remove eight things from your house today and if they are pairs of shoes, that's a definite win!

DAY 9

Now it's time to tackle your underwear drawer. Look through yours and consider how it makes you feel when you wear the items (if you wear them). What do you have that is worn, holey or stained? What can you recycle at a textile

Dispose of your clutter

The biggest issue with having a declutter is always disposing of your former belongings. If you have already planned where it all needs to go, it's essential that you get your discarded items out of your house ASAP. So many of us keep things in the garage or the spare room, or we shove things in the loft and it never ends up going anywhere. During this process, it's vital you clear your home immediately. Hire a man with a van, if necessary, or rope in some willing friends and family to help you. Just don't let it stay in your house for weeks on end. And don't let it sit around in your car, either!

bank? When you feel good from the very first layer of clothes you put on, you'll feel more confident. Perhaps you could ask for some underwear upgrades at Christmas to ensure everything you wear, everything you own, is something that you truly *love* wearing.

DAY 10

At this point, you will have removed a significant amount of stuff and should be feeling clearer in your space. Today, you need to remove 10 items. They don't all need to come from the same category – you can remove an amalgamation of things. What are you going to remove today?

DAY 11

Today, look through your mugs. I know you don't need 20 mugs. *You* know you don't need 20 mugs. Get rid of some! That Sports Direct mug has to go! This is an easy win.

DAY 12

Over the next few weeks, you will continue removing a number of items that correspond with the day

of the challenge. Today, can you get rid of 12 pieces of cutlery or cooking utensils from your kitchen?

A little progress every day adds up to big results.

DAY 13

Children move on from their interests so fast. It's likely you will have many toys that are outgrown, or in which they have lost interest. Trying to rotate toys (see page 93) is a great idea, but at some point you need to admit they need to be removed entirely, either by donating to a toy bank or to a charity shop.

DAY 14

From where can you remove 14 items today? If you have children, look at their baby clothes. It's tempting to keep everything from when they were tiny, but you don't need to keep multiples. The first onesie, the first dress or a special jumper might be enough. See what you can clear out to free up space. I find that keeping multiple items will never spark as much emotion as the very first items do, so it's time to get rid of them.

DAY 15

You've made it halfway through the challenge! Today is your reality check. So far, you will have removed an amazing 120 items from your home, but it's time to reflect on what's left. You will likely still have a lot of stuff (although I'm hoping not too much). Pause a moment to take it in and realise exactly what it is you have donated, what still needs to be sold and what you have kept. Do you still have a huge amount of categories to go through? Or have you done really well and reduced your belongings considerably, maybe even getting rid of more than each day's target? Understand that the items that remain are more than enough and that you don't need to keep buying more. In fact, you didn't need many of the things in the first place. Hopefully, this realisation will finally break the cycle of excessive buying.

Remember, the money you spent on an item is gone. You are not any richer because you store it in your home and you won't be any poorer if you let it go.

DAY 16

Go through ornaments and knick-knacks that clutter your surfaces (and need to be dusted regularly). If there are special pieces given to you by a loved one or items that have an emotional attachment, I'm not suggesting you get rid of them, but look over the objects you have on display and see whether you can edit out less meaningful items, or ones you don't believe to be aesthetically pleasing.

DAY 17

Look at your clothes and consider what you own, compared to what you wear. It's said that we wear just 20% of our wardrobes 80% of the time. The less you have, the easier your laundry loads will be and the less time you'll spend washing, ironing, folding and putting away. What could you do with that free time?! I don't want you to just check your current wardrobe. Check the suitcase of clothes under the bed that you haven't worn since you had a baby and the crate of clothes you wore to work in a job you no longer do. What have you packed away in the loft? Your body shape changes, your lifestyle changes and your personal tastes will change throughout your life. The way you felt about a garment two years ago might not be the same way you feel today. What no longer fits you? What can you store away for another season that will lighten your wardrobe right now? Look at each category of clothes: sportswear, T-shirts, knits, jeans, dresses, skirts... and consider whether you own things in excess. Some people only wear the same clothes on repeat, and if that applies to you, it's time to get rid of everything else by donating it to charity or selling it.

DAY 18

Go through your make-up bags and bathroom cabinets today. Do you have old make-up that has expired? Nail varnish with just a crusty drop in the bottom of the bottle? Are there jars you used once and never went back to? Always use up what you have before you buy something new and keep your products as streamlined as possible. It's time to stop overbuying. For a start, your skin can only handle so many products before it begins to react. What excess items do you have that you can recycle at a high-street chemists? What could you donate to a beauty bank?

DAY 19

I recommend that you look through your books today. What have you read that you won't go back to, what books did you buy that you will never end up reading? What could you share with a friend? What could you donate to a school or library? Can you remove 19 books from your house today?

DAY 20

However tidy you keep your house, paperwork somehow builds up. File everything you can into relevant folders and check through old documents to see if you can shred or recycle them. It's recommended that you don't need to keep paperwork for longer than five tax years and I'm sure you will be able to clear piles of papers if you go through your files today.

'Good order is the foundation of all things.'

Edmund Burke

DAY 21

Today, you are removing 21 items. What areas do you still need to tackle? With every bag that you fill up, ask yourself if you would buy that item again. Ask yourself why you bought it in the first place. Think about what you never need to buy again. What did you waste your money on the first time? You need to look at all this stuff and absorb how much you've removed from your life. Thinking about all the things you bought that you didn't need will help ensure you don't have to repeat this process so intensely next time.

DAY 22

I think it's just as important to declutter your digital storage as it is your physical space. Knowing you have thousands of unread emails can be as mentally draining as a stack of unopened mail. What can you delete from your inbox? What mailers can you unsubscribe from? Save and back up any important files on cloud services to clear space and memory on your computer, so it works fast from day to day.

DAY 23

Do you still have piles of DVDs, even though you are signed up to Netflix? Your favourite films can be streamed nowadays, so go through your DVDs and remove them from your house. There are companies that will buy them off you. Investigate the quickest, smoothest way for these 23 items to be taken away.

DAY 24

In the same way that we can stream films, every song you could possibly want to listen to will be available on Spotify, iTunes or Apple Music. Clear out the space that your CDs (or even cassette tapes) are taking up. I've seen people who no longer have a device to play them on who still keep their CDs! As with DVDs, find a company that will buy them off you.

DAY 25

As you reach these higher numbers, it can potentially feel overwhelming. What 25 things can you take out of your house today? By now, you will have realised that half the stuff in your home are things you don't actually need and the other half are things that you don't actually like. You'll be wondering how all of this stuff even fitted into the space! You'll find items you forgot you had and things you don't even remember buying or being given in the first place. This is where the realisation of how much unnecessary stuff you have in your house kicks in and you will understand that changing your space is vital. It is a very hard part of the decluttering process, but you need to get through it. This method also helps you to see where the gaps are – it highlights what is needed. (Rather like the warehouse scenes in *Sort Your Life Out*, you can see exactly what you own and perhaps what is missing.)

DAY 26

You are in the last few days of the challenge. Today, you could look through memory boxes. Our attachment to certain objects changes over time, so it's important to keep returning to these areas and seeing what you can remove.

DAY 27

As we reach the highest numbers, I often joke that people sometimes panic and end up taking 30 plastic bags to the recycling point. However, if you've been storing cardboard boxes 'just in case', they are very valid items to remove. Remember, you don't have to remove 27 things from the same category. Although today, it is vital that you do get rid of 27 items from your home.

DAY 28

Where can you find 28 more objects to remove? Is it time to go through your kitchen cupboards and remove foodstuffs? What is out of date? What do you have duplicates of, cluttering up your cupboards so everything topples out when you open them? What can you donate to a food bank to make your shelves feel empty, clear and calm?

Small efforts lead to big rewards.

DAY 29

Today, look at seasonal items. Get up in the loft and go through your Easter decorations, Christmas baubles and Halloween novelties. What will you never use again? What are you tired of? It's easy to pick up a few cute decorations and it's tempting to update a festive theme, but we go through so many phases of taste, you're bound to have pieces that you can donate to free up your space.

DAY 30

Have a final check through all your rooms to see what you can remove today. Once you have found 30 final items, you have completed the challenge.

'Happiness is a place between too little and too much.'

Finnish proverb

CONGRATULATIONS!

You've made it! You have achieved the mammoth task of decluttering 465 items from your home.

Hopefully, your space is now feeling lighter and clearer, and you feel like a weight has been lifted off your shoulders. Each room should only contain what you love and what you need.

At the end of this challenge, the most important thing is to be aware of the items that you've removed, so you never go and buy them again. You should now understand the reasons why you have been overbuying and cluttering up your space.

By now, you should be able to stop and think more clearly before you bring anything new, in any category, into your home in the future. You want to keep the space fresh and empty, so don't be tempted to fill it all up with clutter again!

7-DAY SEASONAL CHALLENGE

As well as an annual (or more regular) 30-day challenge, it's essential to keep on top of your home with these seasonal resets. Our moods and our lifestyles change throughout the year and undertaking a 7-day seasonal challenge will give you a gentle boost as the year turns.

Following my decluttering advice will not only give a seasonal boost to your mood, it will allow you to feel calmer, more organised and ready to tackle the season ahead, whatever it holds.

Everyone's home will be different and I want these seasonal resets to benefit *you* and your home, but I have listed and described key actions I believe will help *every* home in *every* season.

In addition to the actions suggested, I would also encourage you to follow the principles of the 30-day challenge and remove an increasing number of objects from your space each day. Even doing this smaller challenge will see you take 28 items out of your home in a week, which is a hugely positive step.

Before you start

tip

Spring

Begin with a space audit (see page 20). Grab a notepad and pen and walk out of your front door, locking it behind you.

Take a few steps back and look at where you live. Take it in and appreciate the value of the space behind your front door, however messy it might have become.

Now unlock the door and walk back inside. Write down the first things you see that you want to change. Where are the problem areas? Split each page in two and jot down what you love too.

Walk slowly through every room in your house and write down exactly what changes you need to make over the course of the next seven days. Look at your home with fresh eyes and more focus.

This process is designed to clarify the areas that need the most attention. It's vital you do this exercise properly.

DAY 1: Light

For me, the most exciting things about spring are new growth, daffodils, and the return of sunlight. With the longer daylight hours, at last, you will want to let the light into your home. Today, we will look at where the light comes into our homes and where it is blocked. Are you allowing enough light to enter your space? How can you let more light in? To do this, look at the windowsills in every room. Take everything off them, clean the sills and the windows, then re-evaluate what you had piled up on there.

Whatever objects you have taken off your windowsills need to be placed in a large empty space so you can edit them. Did the things that lived there before block the light? Should they be returned to other areas of your house? Do you have a lingering dead cactus or a pot of pens that stopped working months ago? They either get put into their proper place, recycled or donated.

Only put back what you need and what you think looks aesthetically pleasing. Try not to cram too much stuff on your sills, they should never be overloaded.

Now you can appreciate the light streaming in, and it's likely you can actually open the windows at last to let the lovely, fresh, spring air into your home. Fresh air is important for our respiratory systems as well as for refreshing our minds.

PLUS remove 1 object from your space

DAY 2: Bedlinen

Spring is the time to change-over your heavy, cosy winter bedlinen and replace it with fresh, lighter-weight linens. Strip down all the beds and change the sheets. Take your duvets to the laundry for a deep clean and wash the blankets you were snuggling in during the colder months. Go through all your sets of bedding to make sure that everything is in good condition. When you have lovely sheets, it will allow you to get into bed with a feeling of joy every night. I store my bedlinen in sets, so all the pillowcases, bottom sheets and duvet covers match and are slotted into a pillowcase from the set. This keeps everything together and is a neat way to store things.

It also means that you won't ever be searching for a rogue pillowcase when it's time to change your sheets and making the bed is a breeze.

PLUS remove 2 objects from your space

DAY 3: Vacuuming

Now your windows are open and there is fresh air flowing through your home, I recommend you pull out all your heavy furniture and vacuum underneath the bulky pieces. Spring cleaning is a tradition that makes perfect sense as we get rid of dust in our homes and replace it with fresh air and light. Try to get under every bed, every wardrobe and chest of drawers in the bedrooms. Get behind the sofa and take all the cushions off it, vacuuming in-between them. You never know what you might find! Consider what items in your home are rarely moved – now is the time to shift them.

PLUS remove 3 objects from your space

DAY 4: Coat cupboard

If you have an understairs cupboard, over the past few months, it's likely that you will have just been throwing your outdoor clothing in there every day, without much thought. Welly boots, heavy coats, scarves, hats, umbrellas... Now is the time to clear it out. Remove everything, clear and thoroughly clean the space.

Group everything together (so coats go together, boots together, etc.). What has been outgrown or has worn out? What can you recycle, donate or sell? Can you pack these seasonal items away and store them in another space (perhaps the loft)? If not, make sure they are put back in relevant sections and the accessories and footwear are separate, in individual containers.

What if you don't have an understairs cupboard? You can still take the principle of how your hall space (or coat rack) often becomes a dumping ground and clear out somewhere else that you know you constantly put things without thinking. Almost every home will have a drawer of doom full of random items that you have been ignoring: medicine syringes, old train tickets, unsharpened pencils... These can all be recycled or returned to their rightful places.

PLUS remove 4 objects from your space

DAY 5: Paperwork

Even if you don't work from home, I suggest you consider making a dedicated office area for dealing with your paperwork and files. So much is now online – and you can create an organised system for accessing your digital files – but there will still be mail and letters coming into your house weekly, or even daily, adding to the overall clutter. In worst-case scenarios, toppling towers of mail can cover every surface and windowsill, and it's common for people to leave their mail unopened for weeks... even months. This aversion to mail stems from the fact that it's rarely a fun job. Unless it's your birthday, you're likely to be receiving bills, invoices and reminders (asking for money or time), so it's tempting to ignore letters. But having unopened mail in your space is a real drain on your mood. Staying on top of your mail, and creating a space to file anything you need to keep, is an essential step in resetting your space and improving your daily mental health.

PLUS remove 5 objects from your space

DAY 6: Car

I usually focus on clearing space in your house, as this is usually the biggest problem, but in spring it's good to dedicate some time to decluttering your car. My method is to take a plastic bag to the car and put all the rubbish in it, vacuum out the dust and crumbs and wipe down the surfaces. You really don't need to keep much in your car, apart from safety items and your logbook, but one thing I do store in there is my carrier bags, ready for shopping. Don't leave them in the house, where you can easily forget them, but keep them in the boot of your car. I use a cool bag to store them and I don't think you need any more bags than what fits in there. Wet wipes and tissues are also useful to keep in your car, but if you have any other essentials, can you get an organiser or caddy to keep them in, so they are neat and tidy? If you really are struggling to keep your car tidy, is it time to take it to a valet and get it professionally cleaned? If you treat yourself, you may be more likely to keep it clean in future.

PLUS remove 6 objects from your space

DAY 7: Emails

We are all faced with the temptation to bring new objects into our homes every single day, and one of the most regular ways this happens is through a constant stream of marketing emails. Companies know that your head will be turned if they pop into your inbox and offer you a discount. Unsubscribe from all emails that come from companies that you shopped with just once or no longer want to buy from. This is particularly key with clothing companies. It's very rare that you will *need* new clothes and if the time comes when you actually have to replace a worn-out item, you will know what brands to head to, without those constant digital reminders to spend money.

PLUS remove 7 objects from your space

Summer

DAY 1: Wardrobe

I have noticed that when decluttering tasks are not effective, sometimes it's because not enough time has been dedicated to the job. Make sure that you are completely committed. You need to choose a free day to work on your chosen area and then stick to it. Book a day off work, get the kids out of the house if they are going to be a distraction, but you need to focus. Commit to a time and then do the work.

You don't need access to every item of clothing – or accessory – you own *every* day of the year. Instead, editing a capsule wardrobe of 25 pieces you'll wear over the next three months is a brilliant way to declutter your closet and streamline your style. Store out-of-season clothes in a suitcase or plastic crates in the loft.

PLUS remove 1 object from your space

DAY 2: Handbag

Summer is the ideal time to clear out your handbag, as you might be swapping from a heavier leather version to a basket or a bag in a lighter colour or fabric. Start by taking everything out of the bag and give it a good shake to get rid of any dust, loose sweets or raisins. Clean the lining and wipe down the outside so it looks in the best condition possible. Then go through everything that was lurking in there. Go through all your receipts and file the ones that you need to keep (recycle the rest). Do you have any random keys that you don't actually need on your key ring? Go through your reward cards. Do you need them with you every day? There's an app where you can store all your reward cards so you don't need to carry the plastic around with you. Do you have any random toys in your bag that can be returned to your children's playroom? Only carry the absolute essentials in your handbag every day. You will save time by not rummaging around for things in the bottom and you will also have less physical weight to cart around. You will feel more organised and lighter, which is always a bonus.

PLUS remove 2 objects from your space

DAY 3: Windows

You'll have given your windows and sills some attention in your spring challenge, but it's likely that you'll notice the smears and dirt on your windows in the gorgeous summer light, so this is the time to give them another clean. Choose a dry, sunny day and clean the glass inside and out. Keep an eye on the windowsills to make sure none of the clutter you cleared in spring is creeping back and blocking the light, or stopping you actually opening the windows.

PLUS remove 3 objects from your space

DAY 4: Soft furnishings

Today, I'd like you to look at your cushions, curtains and blinds. In winter you snuggled into blankets and drew the curtains early but during summer you're likely to be spending more time outside. You don't need your soft furnishings to cosset you in this season so it's the perfect time to refresh them. Take your curtains down and shake them out, or hoover them while they're up. If they are looking past their best, take them to be dry-cleaned for a refresh. Dust your blinds, particularly slatted ones, and dust over your ceilings and skirting boards too. Look at the volume of cushions in your house. Cushions are a lovely way to bring your personality to a room but do you have too many? Could you remove some of them? Take the covers off all your cushions and wash them. Wash the inner pads too, if you can.

PLUS remove 4 objects from your space

DAY 5: Rugs

Following on from the soft furnishings we looked at yesterday, turn your attention to the rugs in your house. Some rugs are now machine washable so, after giving them a hoover, can you pop them in your washing machine (or a larger machine at the laundrette)? If you can't clean them yourself, hire a carpet cleaner or get a specialist rug company to do it for you. While you're cleaning all your soft furnishings, work out if there are any items that you no longer use – or like. Now your rugs are clean, consider whether they still suit the room they're in or whether they make the space look smaller. If they aren't working, it's time to get rid!

PLUS remove 5 objects from your space

DAY 6: Chairs

It's always important to remove the largest problem objects every season, as these will make the biggest impact on your room, letting you see the space for what it could be. Today I'd like you to look at your chairs and stools, both in the kitchen and living areas. Do you use them all? How many do you have? Dispose of any you just don't need.

PLUS *remove 6 objects from your space*

DAY 7: Suitcases

As our minds often turn to travel and holidays during the summer months, it's the ideal time to look at your suitcases and travel bags. I find most people store their cases in the loft, so bring them all down and look over them to make sure they're still in good enough condition to use. Do the zips close? Do the wheels work? Are there cracks or splits that could get worse on one more journey? If you decide they're not good enough to use this summer, find out where you could donate or sell them. It will be easy to move them on, as many people will also be travelling and might be in need of cases. With the ones you're keeping, wipe them down and dust out the linings, so they are fresh and clean when you come to pack them. I find storing smaller cases inside larger ones saves space.

PLUS *remove 7 objects from your space*

Autumn

DAY 1: Chimney

As the nights draw in and it gets ever colder, it's time to prepare for harsher weather. As you start your seasonal autumn refresh, get your chimney swept, if you have an open fire. It's necessary to get rid of any residual soot in your chimney for safety and hygeine, and will make every winter fire even warmer.

PLUS remove 1 object from your space

Let the falling autumn leaves remind you just how beautiful it is to declutter.

DAY 2: Toys

If you have children, it's likely they are spending more time playing inside. Now is a great time to bring some structure to their playroom, if they have one, or the area where they store their toys. You'll have made a dent in this if you completed the Dolly Dash in Part Three, but take the time now to give this your full attention.

When I go into a playroom, I empty it completely – all the toys are removed into separate piles, in a different room where possible. Look at the space in the room and consider whether you could change it around to work better for you. Do you need to add more storage or reduce the storage depending on what you're keeping? Arrange all the toys by type. Group each category together and put them into suitable storage containers. Add labels to everything, so every member of the household knows where objects should be put back when not in use.

PLUS remove 2 objects from your space

DAY 3: Cookware

In summer, it's easy to put together a meal with cold food from the fridge, but autumn is definitely the time we start to cook more. We crave hot food: stews, roasts, puddings... Set aside a couple of hours to go through your baking trays, roasting dishes, ovenware and saucepans and ensure they're in the best condition, particularly if you will be entertaining over the colder months. It's also a good idea to check over your slow cooker, if you use one, or any other gadgets and appliances (ensure you are only keeping those you actually use – not the pasta machine you bought, used once and then never looked at again). While you're decluttering your cookware, you could also give your oven a deep clean, or book an oven-cleaning company to do it for you, so it's sparkling fresh before the festive season.

PLUS remove 3 objects from your space

DAY 4: Batteries

Right now is the ideal time to look at your batteries. Take any expired ones to be recycled and update your storage to ensure you always have the right battery to hand. It's particularly useful to do this in autumn as you might be adding fairy lights to your decor, or your children might be playing with more toys inside that need batteries. I think the best way to store them is in a dedicated battery organiser (you can find them online), so you know that all the batteries in that organiser are brand new and you're not second guessing whether they're functional or not, which always leads to stress and annoyance! Battery organisers also let you see exactly what you have, so you know when you're

running out of a certain type. This will also stop you overbuying.

PLUS remove 4 objects from your space

DAY 5: Arts and crafts

Declutter your arts, crafts and hobby items. There are several charities, including pensforkids.co.uk, that will take away all your used pens, crayons, pencils and felt tips that you no longer use, so you can clear out pen pots and get rid of random pencils lurking in drawers.

PLUS remove 5 objects from your space

DAY 6: Magazines

Magazines pile up fast, so now is the time to give them one more flick through, save anything you want to keep, and recycle those you're finished with. You could see if any friends or family would like to read them before you recycle them. This is also a good time to consider whether you really need all the magazines you buy. If you have a subscription, is it time to cancel it? Do you tear open the wrapping every month or let the new issue languish with your other unopened mail? You're in control of what comes into your house every month, so make sure, if you keep subscribing, that you will read each issue.

PLUS remove 6 objects from your space

DAY 7: Gutters

Once the leaves have finished falling, it's time for you to clear out your gutters. Leaves will block gutters and cause leaks and potential damp in your home. It's time to do it now before the real cold weather sets in and you move into hibernation mode. Sweep paths of any leaves too, so they don't get slippery and become dangerous.

Consider what other areas outside your house you could declutter. Is there a trampoline that never gets used? Do you have kids' bikes that are outgrown? I often use Facebook Marketplace or Freecycle to find out if there is someone local who could take them off my hands.

Use this time to check over your garden furniture before you pack it away or cover it up for winter. Check if anything is broken or beyond repair. If it is, it's time to get rid of it!

PLUS remove 7 objects from your space

Winter

DAY 1: Clothes

During the coldest part of the year, our thoughts turn to comfort and cosiness. When we are at home we want to batten down the hatches against the weather and feel snug. Changing into a fluffy tracksuit when you come inside from the chill can be an excellent way to help you switch off and unwind, so today it's time to go through your loungewear and slippers. What is in worn condition that doesn't make you feel good when you wear it? What do you own multiples of, which could be pared down? Have you got a dressing gown that is past its best, but could be donated? Or if it's in too bad a condition, take it to be recycled at a textile bank. Are your slippers fluffy and snug?

PLUS remove 1 object from your space

DAY 2: Appliances

Change the filters in your household appliances. Your washing machine, dishwasher and vacuum cleaner will all need to have their filters cleaned out periodically. You'll be amazed at how much lint and dirt has gathered in them. What other appliances do you have in your home that you could give a thorough clean, to ensure they run smoothly and work to their best over the coming months?

PLUS remove 2 objects from your space

DAY 3: Hot beverages

I love a good cup of tea or coffee, and taking time to create a neat, clean hot drinks station in your kitchen will make prepping a simple cuppa a pleasure. Go through your coffee pods, beans or bags – however you take it – and make sure it's stored in a container. Get rid of anything out of date. Likewise, with teabags. Store each type of bag in a separate container. Check through your cupboards too. Do you have any random tea flavours you thought you liked the sound of, and never drank again? Get rid! In a composter, if you have one. Now is also time to descale your coffee machine and your kettle to ensure they run efficiently during the winter months (when you're likely to be drinking more hot beverages).

PLUS remove 3 objects from your space

*Detox not just clutter,
but negative emotions,
toxic friendships and
relationships.*

DAY 4: Negative influences

Detoxing the negative energy that surrounds us can make a huge impact on our behaviour, our routines and the way that we feel. Are your friends and family supportive or do they constantly offload their negative thoughts and opinions onto you? Perhaps you have that one friend who rings you every day just to moan. Maybe there are friends who tell you that you will never achieve your goals. They dumb down your ideas or make fun of your choices. Today it's time to reduce the impact they have on you.

Without realising, we also spend a lot of time absorbing negativity from sources all around us. Television programmes that are all about doom and gloom... Shows that boast unrealistic ways of living... Flashy series that make our lives feel lesser somehow... Social media accounts that show us curated lives that seem unachievable. It's great to have opportunities for escapism, but sometimes that escape starts making real life seem worse. Watching *The Kardashians* can be great, but if you watch too much, you'll suddenly feel like you're not achieving your goals or missing out (unless you live in a mansion in LA...).

Write a list of the people in your group of friends who give you the most joy – as well as those that you find hard to be around. Who do you want to see more of? Who do you want to see less of? As you go through the season, jot down the amount of times you see each person. Arrange to see the people that make you happiest. The time you spend with positive influences should definitely outweigh those negative people. Make sure you don't give any more than 10% of your time to those that don't give you joy.

I'm not suggesting that you have to completely edit people or things out of your life, but do think about reducing the time that you let them be around you, or how you are influenced by them. You deserve to be surrounded by people who support you, nourish you and love you. Likewise, social media accounts can be muted or unfollowed, to allow you some breathing space.

PLUS remove 4 objects from your space

DAY 5: Mattress

Today I would suggest that you look at your mattresses. It's time to strip your bed, hoover your mattress, flip it over and make sure it's still giving you proper support. It's advisable to change your mattress every 10 years – is yours overdue an update?

PLUS remove 5 objects from your space

DAY 6: Pillows

Look at your pillows. The feeling of sinking into new pillows can't be beaten, so check that yours are still plump, fluffy and clean. You can wash synthetic pillows in the machine or take feather ones to the laundrette to refresh. Consider using padded pillow protectors, which will help prolong their life. Replace any pillows that are flat and yellow.

PLUS remove 6 objects from your space

DAY 7: Christmas

For most families, the biggest event of winter is usually Christmas, which comes with all the decorations and potential clutter attached. I store all my Christmas decorations in clear containers so I can see what is in each one, as well as labelling them clearly, too. I separate garlands and lights and make sure my lights are divided into further small containers. Each container has a different group of lights within and they never go back tangled up!

When it's time to put your Christmas decorations away, choose somewhere that isn't easy to access. You won't need to use them for the next 11 months, so if you have a loft, I'd suggest putting them in there.

It's a good idea to put away your seasonal decorations in order. The next ones you're likely to use are Easter, followed by Halloween. Each time you put those decorations away, move them to the furthest point, so the next festive decos are the closest to you.

PLUS remove 7 objects from your space

FINAL WORDS

Changing your mindset over your space can be so beneficial. I've seen the effects so many times during my career. From the days when I just worked in private homes through to the experience with my mum's house in Somerset, the basis of the business that I've built and the reason that I am now teaching you about organisation is that I have lived and worked through every type of organisational experience you can imagine.

The biggest moment of change for me was being able to help my mum. I want to help you, too. Even the smallest changes can create happiness in a space in just a few moments. It's so simple to make the beds, put things away in order, or make space to prepare tea and coffee without knocking over a pile of mugs first.

But your home will not change unless *you* are ready to change. It will not stay pristine unless *you* keep up with a constant journey of decluttering. Changing your space can only come from changing your mindset and that's down to *you*.

This book should have given you enough tools to change your space on a practical level. Remember how you want your life to continue and remember that there's no one else that can force you to change. You just have to be ready.

Are you ready?

Dilly x

USEFUL RESOURCES

TRAINING COURSE

After spending 20 years as a professional organiser, I decided to create a fully accredited course to help other people on their journey to become an independent professional organiser. How successful you become is down to the effort you put in. Nothing worth doing comes easily.

Over a 12-week period, I host weekly one-to-ones where I share my tips on how to start and grow your business. It's not an easy process. I am honest with you from day one and anyone who joins my course will be required to put in a lot of hard work and dedication.

The course will test your commitment and effort to better yourself each week, with the goal of giving you the ability to work full-time as a professional organiser, if you are able to commit fully to the job.

To find out more, and to sign up, visit: mailchi.mp/685988a55ef5/waitinglist

STORAGE PRODUCTS & RESOURCES

Some of the essential kit I use is listed below, but please do not go on a storage shopping spree before you have planned out exactly what you need. You will end up buying more than you require, which in turn means you'll have more unused stuff cluttering up your house again!

> Baskets

> Drawer dividers

> Dyno label maker

> Kilner jars

> Lazy Susans

> Food containers (stackable)

> Large lidded storage boxes

> Make-up organisers/trays

> Slimline velvet hangers

> Heavy-duty clothes rail

> Rail protectors

You can shop my favourite products directly from my Declutter Dollies Store on Amazon, along with iDesign and Wham World.

www.amazon.co.uk/shop/dclutterdollies

www.idesignlivesimply.com/uk-en

www.whatmoreuk.com

Notes

Notes

Notes

_____

_____

_____

_____

_____

_____

_____

_____

_____

_____

_____

_____

_____

_____

_____

_____

Notes

Notes

Notes

Notes

_____
_____
_____
_____
_____
_____
_____
_____
_____
_____
_____
_____
_____
_____
_____
_____
_____

Notes

_____

_____

_____

_____

_____

_____

_____

_____

_____

_____

_____

_____

_____

_____

_____

_____

Notes

Notes

Notes